Ask the Chiropractor

Ask the Chiropractor

Steven J. Pollack, D.C.

iUniverse, Inc.
New York Lincoln Shanghai

Ask the Chiropractor

iUniverse, Inc.

For information address:
iUniverse, Inc.
2021 Pine Lake Road, Suite 100
Lincoln, NE 68512
www.iuniverse.com

ISBN: 0-595-32404-5 (pbk)
ISBN: 0-595-66554-3 (cloth)

Printed in the United States of America

I dedicate my second book of "Ask the Chiropractor" to the founding fathers of Chiropractic. They sacrificed their lives for a conviction to a science, art and philosophy that was well before their age. These great leaders were mavericks of a noble cause that was not understood. The essence and purity of their actions enabled present and future Chiropractors. As they paved the road to a new-fashioned magical healing art, they put themselves against all the odds of survival. Our founding Chiropractic brethren committed to educating the public masses that Chiropractic is the mainstream primary care necessary for natural healing in all human beings. Only truthful universally intelligent theories exist over the length of time. Now, in the new millenium, humanity seeks what these great men perceived more than 100 years ago. A paradigm shift has occurred in the mindset of mankind. Above-down-inside-out is where we come from and how we heal. Knowledge is power and while humanity is seeking the answers to life and health now is the premier time to engage the populace with the ideals of Chiropractic. My Chiropractic forefathers who unconditionally and with endless energy, passionately believed in their dream inspire this book and my career.

Contents

How to benefit from these columns

I. Public relations

1. Start your own column in local papers.

    a. Make your face familiar to the public.

    b. Repetition sells in marketing

2. Reference columns for patient education.

    a. Save time in explanation. Time for more patients.

    b. Educate your staff.

3. Open doors by validating yourself as an established professional in the community.

    a. Use columns in mailings.

    b. Use columns in portfolio to obtain lectures and events in your community.

4. Education of your community, friends, family, and employees.

5. Web-site promotions and E-mail lists.

II. Personal growth

A. Create your own question and answer columns besides existing questions and answers in this book.

B. Stay in touch with everything happening in the Chiropractic profession.

C. Express yourself. Be heard by thousands in your community.

D. Maintain your philosophical beliefs.

E. Increase listening skills to grasp new ideas and questions on health from patients, employees, friends, and family.

III. Our profession

A. Your time is a gift back to the profession.

B. Expand the circle of knowledge. Inspire new well-grounded students of Chiropractic.

Adjustments may ease menopause symptoms

Question: I was stunned recently to read in the *New York Times* that hormone replacement was more dangerous than helpful. The article didn't give alternatives to the therapy. What could you suggest as an alternative to hormone-replacement therapy for women?

Answer: I am very aware of the article and news releases regarding the dangers of hormone-replacement therapy. The in-depth study discovered that drugs, a combination of estrogen and progestin caused small increases in breast cancer, heart attacks, strokes and blood clots. Those risks outweighed the drugs' benefits, a small decrease in hip fractures and a decrease in colorectal cancer.

The study, supported by the National Institutes of Health, sent letters to many of the 16,000 women in the study, telling them to discontinue the drugs in light of the results.

A large concern of many women is the consequences of suddenly stopping. To answer this question and your question regarding alternatives, let us examine why these drugs are given in the first place.

Until recently, medical authorities were telling doctors to encourage almost every woman to start taking hormone-replacement drugs when she reached menopause, and to take them for years, even for life. Their purpose was to reduce the natural side effects that come with some women's menopause, including night sweats, embarrassing hot flashes, moodiness, and depression. The most common reason doctors encouraged the drug regime was to prevent osteoporosis, which is a progression of demineralization of bone tissue.

Considering the symptoms the drug regimes intended to correct, we have found that there can be coinciding or other causes of these side effects. Nutritionally, it has been demonstrated that supplementation of the appropriate amount of calcium-magnesium in the diet as well as vitamin E has been successful in combating the menopausal symptoms. A proper diet, avoiding caffeinated beverages and high-sugar concentrated products, supports natural progression through menopause.

Chiropractically, we have a lot of success when neurological disturbed energy flow to the reproductive area is corrected through adjustments to the pelvis and lumbar spine.

You can't stop Mother Nature, but you can assist her in natural progression through what can be a difficult time for some women. If you have severe or persistent symptoms, you should absolutely consult your own physician before replacing or stopping drug treatment.

Quote of the week: *"If there's a way to do it better...find it."*—Thomas Edison

Animals can receive Chiropractic adjustments

Question: My golden retriever has been limping since a car hit him. Can Chiropractors treat a dog's hip problems like the one my dog has?

Answer: Animals get excellent results with Chiropractic adjustments and have been for many years. In the state of New Jersey it is required that a Chiropractor that treats animals also has a Veterinarian license. There are not many Chiropractors with dual degrees, but they can be contacted. Many of these specialized Chiropractors treat horses. There is a rigid control on racehorses and what chemicals or drugs can be administered to them. When a horse is sick or injured even medication to assist their health will be demonstrated in a blood test. The positive testing for a drug could eliminate a horse's qualifications to compete. It is for this reason that a natural healing approach is utilized to assist and promote health in these competitive animals. The same holds true for racing greyhounds and other competitive show dogs. Qualified Chiropractors are also common working with livestock on farms, more so out west. It makes sense that if a high-profile animal receives the best natural care to maintain its health, then why shouldn't your family loved pet also receive that same quality care?

I have personally had three golden retrievers as pets and find that it is imperative to keep their hips aligned. Larger breeds of dogs do have tendencies to develop or be genetically inclined to hip dysplasia or hip arthritis as they mature. In the case of a trauma such as your dog's car accident it is very important to get to your personal Veterinarian as soon as possible to examine your pet. Pets can't always communicate the extent of their injuries with just postural and behavioral habit changes. A trained professional should carefully examine your pet to determine potential internal injuries or life threatening damage.

A responsible pet owner should always observe their animal for consistent changes in normal behavior, feed their animal natural healthy diets, exercise their animal, and give them plenty of water and even more love.

Quote of the week: *"No man is a failure who is enjoying life."*—William Feather

Exercise caution with antibiotics

Question: When should I give my child antibiotics?

Answer: Your question is a very good considering the confusion amidst many health professionals and other parents. A study published in the journal *Pediatrics* in February 2003 surveyed 200 families with children between the ages of 6 months and 5 years and found that many parents do not know basic information about colds and their lack of knowledge can lead to dangerous mistakes.

While a majority of the parents (93 percent) understood that colds are caused by viruses, 66 percent also thought bacteria was the cause. Unfortunately, over half of the parents (53 percent) believed that children with colds need antibiotics: 23 percent believed that the child needs to go to the emergency room, and 60 percent thought that a visit to the child's doctor was in order.

Antibiotics do not work on viruses and incorrect use can lead to antibiotic-resistant bacteria. Here is what the Academy of Pediatrics wants parents to know:

1. There is no cure for the common cold.

2. Children with colds breathe through their mouths, which dries the mouth and throat, so the child should be given a lot of water and fruit juice.

3. Support your child with natural wholesome foods with nutrients.

4. Use a clean, cool mist humidifier in your child's room. (Adding a half-cup of apple cider vinegar to the water is helpful also.)

5. Monitor your child's temperature and check on them regularly.

6. Don't give antibiotics or over-the-counter medications.

7. Don't give aspirin to a child because it can cause Reye's syndrome.

8. Caution should only be taken if the child develops trouble breathing, has a cold for longer than 10 days, has a fever over 101 degrees or fever that lasts longer than two days, or if ear or throat pain becomes severe. Then a doctor visit is warranted.

Quote of the week: *"There are really only three kinds of people: those who make things happen, those who watch things happen, and those who say, "What happened?""*—unknown author

Arthritis pains at night are common

Question: I am very active in my daily activities between work and athletics. During the day I feel fine but in the morning my joints get achy and inflamed. Why does this occur?

Answer: You are describing a common occurrence with rheumatoid inflammatory response. When you are active and mobile with your joints the natural motion transfers fluids across your joint surfaces, lubricating and dispensing toxic by-products by natural breakdown. Conditions of chondromalacia (joint deterioration) surface damage such as in knee meniscus damage, vertebral disc compression, scar tissue and general degeneration minimize joint functions and proper lubrication. As long as you stay active and move all your joints daily you will minimize joint pain and dysfunction throughout the day. When you become sedentary or when you sleep it is a natural mechanism of the body to attract fluid to irritated tissues of the body. Your condition may be a joint surface problem. Once you are at rest the joint surface will increase its temperature which is normal. The body senses increased temperature change and responds by trying to neutralize it with fluids filled with minerals, vitamins, and enzymes. The accumulation of these fluids on the joint surface while at rest is considered a rheumatoid arthritic response. Osteoarthritis, which is bony irritation, can produce a similar response, only it occurs more while motion is occurring.

Chiropractic adjustments of improperly aligned joint positions, along with proper nutrition and exercise can correct many of these conditions or at least minimize discomfort.

Quote of the week: *"He can who thinks he can, and he can't who thinks he can't. This is an inexorable, indisputable law."*—Orison Swett Marden

Baby's sleep interruption may be behavioral

Question: My 5-month-old hasn't been sleeping through the night. She gets up three to four times a night. We feel like we have tried everything our pediatrician suggested without success. Could something be wrong with her? Are there any procedures in Chiropractic that may help?

Answer: Infant sleep disorders are very common. I will first always suggest you continue your communication and relationship with your pediatrician considering he is familiar with your baby.

My suggestions are based on my experience with sleep disorders in children in general. I find that a good amount of the disorders are due to new parents being overly sensitive. Many infants will get fussy and must learn to go back to sleep on their own. When a parent cuddles or attends to the baby at every whimper, the parent may be conditioning the behavior and feeding the condition rather than correcting it. It takes courage to listen to your child cry or whimper and not attend to them. Some experts feel that cutting back each night to the number of times and amount of time you attend to the baby can initiate appropriate sleeping patterns.

A mom or dad usually knows the difference between a serious cry or overtired whine. Most parents will tell you they were able to handle their second child much easier than their first.

Many other causes can affect infant sleep. Colic can disturb digestion. We find that colic is commonly an allergy to their formula or a reaction to their mother's breast milk from eating an irritable food.

Upper cervical subluxations are common in children. Childbirth is a very traumatic event in a newborn's life. Commonly, the first two vertebras in the neck can be misaligned, interfering with proper nerve supply to the tissues and organs of the head and upper body. Correction with very gentle specific adjustments by a Chiropractor has successfully treated these subluxations and directly affected infant sleep interruptions positively.

Any persistent symptom or excessive activity of a child that stays unresolved for weeks should always be attended to by a professional child health-care provider.

Quote of the week: *"When you do not know what you are doing and what you are doing is the best, that's inspiration."*—Robert Bresson

Baby walkers are dangerous

Question: Are baby walkers safe for my baby?

Answer: There is an extremely high risk of injury with the use of baby walkers with young children. The amount of evidence indicating this is accumulating. In 1999, in the United States 8,800 children under the age of 15 months were treated in emergency rooms from baby walker injuries. The most common cause of injuries resulted from falls downs stairs, subsequently injuring the head.

The scary part of these statistics is that the majority of these injuries occurred while a caretaker was in the room with the child in the walker. The committee on Injury and Poison Prevention of the American Academy of Pediatrics gave other reasons to ban baby walkers. Walkers do not help an infant to learn how to walk, and can delay normal motor and mental development.

From my perspective of treating children for 22 years, baby walkers are dangerous to appropriate pelvic development by putting weight bearing on structures not ready to bear weight. They also prevent proper cross crawl gait function, which allows the brain body co-ordination to develop. When a baby lifts its opposing arm and leg up alternating left then right it stimulates the brain to prepare for proper walking. Walkers bypass this important part of the instinctual education to the child and may disrupt brain development as well as coordination.

Let nature take its course. Please don't use walkers as temporary babysitters. You can love and enjoy your child more without walkers.

Quote of the week: *"Anything in life that we don't accept will simply make trouble for us until we make peace with it."*—Shakti Gawain

Booster seats prevent injuries in accidents

Question: What type of safety belt will protect my 6-year-old's spine if we were to get into an auto accident?

Answer: Unfortunately there is no seat belt that prevents or gives total protection from auto accidents. Even the slightest fender bender transfers unnatural forces to the spine. A study published by the *Journal of the American Medical Association* researched 3,616 accidents involving 4,243 children in 15 states and found that children in booster seats suffered injuries in 0.77 percent of crashes, compared to 1.95 percent of children who were using seat belts only. None of the children in booster seats suffered from spinal cord or abdominal injuries, whereas injuries in children using seat belts included all parts of their body.

Booster seats that correctly position seat belts should be required for all children up to the age of 7 based on research from the Children's Hospital of Philadelphia. Maine is the only state that requires booster seats up to the age of 8.

The parent or guardian of a child under 8 can maintain additional protection and prevention by checking strap positions for snugness and proper placement prior to driving. Utilization of a soft material over the seat belt can supply comfort to your child also.

Should you have the misfortune of being in a motor vehicle accident you should have your spine checked first by a Chiropractor, no matter how light you may feel the impact or the damage may have been. The physics of impact between two 2-ton objects colliding at any speed transfers enormous forces to a 50 to 200 pound object, meaning you. The body, especially the spine, does not always exhibit symptoms from these impacts immediately. In fact, many patients do not exhibit symptoms until weeks or even months after the initial accident. The earlier appropriate treatment is administered the less likely your injuries will be symptomatic as well as severe. Many times parents do not consider their children in an accident because they don't complain. Young children do not have the ability to decipher severity of injury nor can they communicate specifically the location of their symptoms. Any spinal injury is a deep concern because with or without symptoms it can affect spinal growth and development.

If you or someone you know is in an automobile accident with their children make sure they all get checked by a Chiropractor as soon as possible.

Quote of the week: *"Success means we go to sleep at night knowing that our talents and abilities were used in a way that served others."*—Marianne Williamson

Breast-feeding is best for mother and baby

Question: While I was pregnant I was given some formula products and the literature to go with them. I chose not to breast-feed my newborn based on that information. I am sorry I did not breast-feed because I now know many of the great benefits of nursing. Would you please tell other new moms in your column what I found out too late?

Answer: Expectant mothers should be cautioned about the influence of baby formula advertisements according to many studies. Mothers who were given formula-company literature, as reviewed in one study, were five times more likely to stop breast-feeding the first few days following delivery.

This is a crime in my opinion because that infant's natural immunity is enhanced with his or her mom's colostrum in the first six weeks of life.

I will just list some of the benefits of breast-feeding:

- It enhances the deep emotional relationship between mother and baby.

- It produces better social and emotional development of the baby, produces a better psychomotor development, allows better growth and helps faster recovery from illness.

- It satisfies the suckling mechanism of the baby, diminishes frequency of baby's tooth cavities, prevents the development of pathogenic germs in the intestines, diminishes the possibilities of infant colic, diabetes, obesity, ear infections, allergic illness and diaper rash.

- Breast-feeding also assists the mother by diminishing the incidence of breast and ovarian cancer, puerperal bleeding, depression and osteoporosis.

- Other benefits include saving money and time; offering a more hygienic and sterile method of feeding that contains all the nutrients your infant will need; diminishing the use of medications; preventing environmental pollution; diminishing a tendency toward child abuse and frequency of newborn abandonment.

There is nothing more natural than a mother breast-feeding her child. For more information contact the La Leche League.

Quote of the week: *"Life is not measured by the number of breaths we take, but by the moments that take our breath away."*—author unknown

Boost your immune system

Question: I have not been able to get rid of the flu this year. I think I am getting better then the flu symptoms return again. What can you suggest to help me get rid of the flu once and for all?

Answer: Yes, this year's flu seems to be affecting more people than ever and the symptoms are stronger and more prolonged. Prevention is the best policy, but that won't help you at this point. How you treat the flu once you get it is based on your belief system in health care. I will give you the natural approach that we suggest to our families and patients.

First, I suggest you boost your immune system with supplemental anti-oxidants such as vitamin C as well as zinc and calcium. Herbal remedies containing Echinacea, golden seal and chamomile can be supportive also. There are many choices and combinations of cold remedies available. Herbal teas are also very effective. Always consult a specialist in nutrition to find the best supplementation for you as an individual.

What you delete from your dietary intake is as important as what you add when it comes to boosting your immune system. Minimize caffeine, sugar, salt; dense carbohydrates such as rice potatoes, pasta and bread, and most importantly eliminate dairy products that cause mucous formation. Drinking plenty of water and clear broth fluids is essential to prevent dehydration secondary to fevers. Apple cider vinegar is an excellent detoxification agent that can be gargled with. It can also be used in a hot-air humidifier during sleep to break up congestion. Fresh lemons and lemon juice can be used in the same way.

Identify any stress in your life that is presently diminishing your quality of life. If possible, confront your stress at home, work or in your relationships. Harboring pent-up stress lowers the immune system drastically. Find a safe outlet to break up your stress and laugh a lot. When you feel ill changing your state of mind can work wonders for healing.

Chiropractic is an outstanding method of assisting the immune system to fight flu conditions. Chiropractors help balance the nervous system, which directly controls the immune system. When patients tell us they can't make it in to our office due to having the flu we encourage them to get in—especially on these days to help them heal more efficiently. The patients that do are very grateful.

The final ingredient to fighting the flu is plenty of rest. Help your body to help itself.

Quote of the week: *"Have the courage to act instead of react."—Earlene Larson Jenks*

Check car seats for child's safety

Question: I was recently in a car accident with my children sitting in the backseat. My children were jolted even with the safety harness on. Could my children have suffered injuries? Could I have prevented the injuries?

Answer: Car seat safety is a priority issue in the present state of society. Children are being transported to school, sporting events, music, ballet, and pretty much everywhere on a daily basis. Children spend hours in vehicles daily. Safety is imperative whether you are a cautious driver or not. It is usually the other guy that creates the accident.

According to Stephanie Tombrello, executive director of Safety Belt Safe USA, "If after you've tightened your child into his or her car seat, you can still pinch the fabric of the harness straps between your fingers, the harness is to loose."

The danger posed on a child with a loose harness is that he or she can easily come out of their car seat in a crash. The child could then be severely injured if he hits part of the cars interior or another passenger. The worst case scenario; the child is ejected from the vehicle altogether.

The majority of fender benders do not eject the child out of their seat. The child can be jolted forward then backward rapidly creating a whiplash phenomenon. Many adults do not consider the child in a motor vehicle accident. If the adult suffered a whiplash injury in the accident then the odds are very high that the children did also. All children of all ages should be checked by a Chiropractor immediately after auto accidents. Many symptoms do not appear right away. A Chiropractor can detect and help correct injuries sustained to your child in an auto accident. The sooner you bring them in the less chance of irritation and scar tissue development.

To avoid injury to your children tighten the harness straps-so they are snug and have no slack. In the case of an accident, get to your family Chiropractor as soon as possible.

Quote of the week: *"It is a funny thing about life; if you refuse to accept anything but the best, you very often get it."*—Somerset Maugham

Chiropractic can correct CTS

Question: I work at a computer and everyone at my job says they have carpal tunnel. What is it and can Chiropractors correct it?

Answer: Carpal tunnel is actually called carpal tunnel syndrome (CTS), and it is the name given to the symptoms that occur when the nerves and blood vessels running through the carpal tunnel in the wrist are compressed, causing swelling and inflammation of those nerves (median nerves).

The tunnel is formed by the connection of two of your wrist bones by a band of ligament tissue. Overuse or swelling onto the median nerve leads to pain, weakness and other associated CTS symptoms.

Many patients describe the pain as being worse at night, even waking them out of their sleep. The pain can also radiate up the arm and to the back of the shoulder.

The U.S. Department of Labor called CTS the chief occupational hazard of the 1990s. It affects more than 8 million Americans and accounts for more than 50 percent of work-related injuries.

The causes of CTS vary from work related to recreational activities. Like you, long hours on the keyboard with improper had positioning and posture can lead to CTS. Other common causes include: grasping a steering wheel too tightly, repetitive use of vibrating tools and any activity that puts the wrist in consistently awkward positions.

Recreational causes include weight lifting, cycling and rowing as well as crafts such as needlework and weaving. Other conditions can mimic CTS and must be ruled out including diabetes, alcoholism, arthritis, gout fractures, spinal problems, hypothyroidism and pregnancy.

Chiropractors can determine if you are a good candidate for correction by taking a good history, checking your ranges of motion, strength, neurological integrity and performing other diagnostic tests if necessitated.

Chiropractic is an approach to health care that is natural, drugless and non-invasive.

If your Chiropractor does not believe that Chiropractic care is the most effective treatment in your individual case, it is the Chiropractor's job to refer you to the next most appropriate health-care professional.

Quote of the week: *"The person that does the things that count usually doesn't stop to count them."*—Anonymous

Chiropractic care can help with fertility

Question: I recently saw a news release on the Internet that Chiropractors can help with fertility. Is this true?

Answer: Yes it is true. Chiropractors can help many cases of people with fertility problems. A recent press release about research into Chiropractic and fertility, distributed by the World Chiropractic Alliance, has generated widespread coverage on television stations around the nation as well as the Internet.

Madeline Behrendt, lead researcher for the series of articles in the *Journal of Vertebral Subluxation Research,* was spotlighted on a special syndicated television news feature.

In the interview Dr. Behrendt made certain the audience understood what Chiropractic was really for.

"The Chiropractor identifies spinal distortions, which are called subluxations, and once they were detected and corrected, the fertility function, improved," she explained.

According to the Centers for Disease Control, more than six million women in the United States are infertile and more than nine million use some kind of infertility service.

Chiropractors correct nerve interference that may be occurring in both partners in a relationship that is attempting to have a child. Identifying this potential assistance through Chiropractic is not a new revelation. Chiropractors not only treat patients with fertility concerns, but also newborns, pregnant moms and children of all ages and have been doing so since the origin of Chiropractic in 1895.

Quote of the week: *"If you don't know where you are going any path will get you there."*—Lewis Carroll

Chiropractic care initially requires frequent visits

Question: I am being treated by a Chiropractor for a neck problem. Initially he wants to see me three times a week and said this is normal protocol for many spinal conditions. Why do these conditions require frequent visits?

Answer: Every patient and every condition is unique. Everyone is exposed to stress on a daily basis. How you adapt to your stress or not adapt to your stress registers with the nervous system. Your central nervous system (CNS), which is harbored by your skull and vertebral bones, permanently stores information as it is exposed to environmental stimuli. Your CNS then sets up patterns and conditioned responses to any similar stimuli that you get exposed to. When the musculo-skeletal system is referring impulses to the CNS it may respond by patterning an excessive or reduced impulse. Either instance demonstrates abhorrent patterns. A real life scenario may be someone that works on an assembly line who constantly is lifting and turning his or her neck and arms the same way hours at a time or someone who sits at a computer improperly, leaning forward and looking off to one side. These repetitive activities produce long-term patterns that create physiological changes. The muscles and ligaments in those people performing these repetitive movements adapt by getting tighter, larger and possible more sensitive. Asymmetry in the body creates malfunctions leading to dis-ease. Many conditions do not demonstrate symptoms at first. A severe trauma such as a whiplash injury in an auto accident may give a person immediate symptoms and create a deep imbedded pattern in the CNS also.

Whether your abhorrent neurological patterns are from an individual episode or from repetitive behaviors, the CNS must be re-educated to its normal healthy patterns in order for health to be restored. Chiropractors specialize in correcting abhorrent activity to the CNS. The adjustments to your spine are far more than a pop or crack that you may hear. The adjustments to your spine are re-educating nerve impulses to restore function to every cell, tissue, and organ in your body. Initially, it is imperative to keep breaking the old patterns and assist the healthy ones. This enables the body to recover. The good news is that your body never forgets the healthy patterns and is driven to maintain its own healthy functional status. The protocol your Chiropractor gave you appears well within the scope of normal practice.

Quote of the week: *"Destiny is not a matter of chance: it is a matter of choice. It is not something to be waited for; but rather something to be achieved."*—William Jennings Bryan

Chiropractic dates back to early civilization

Question: Where does the name "Chiropractic" come from?

Answer: The name "Chiropractic" comes from the Latin-based roots "chiro" which means "hands or hands on" and "practice" which means the "application of or practice of." Chiropractic therefore means, by Latin definition, the practice of putting the hands on. In more modern terms it means the application of the hands on the spine to correct neurological interference.

Chiropractic origins date back as far as the first Egyptian civilizations. While I was traveling in Italy I was amazed by the original Egyptian hieroglyphics at a museum. One block of these ancient picture writings denoted a spine with arrows extending away from the spine to various body parts and body organs. The museum curator interpreted the writings for me and described the pictures to mean that the spine controlled all the functions of the body including the organs, and that the Egyptians did healings through the spine to help these specific structures. These interpretations are still the basis of modern Chiropractic today.

From Hippocrates (the Father of Medicine) and Galen (the Prince of Physicians) to the 1st century bonesetters of the British Isles, many great men recognized the importance of the spine and nervous system as they relate to the health of the individual.

Today, with our increased knowledge and technology comes an appreciation for natural conservative health-care methods as viable alternatives. Chiropractic offers the "holistic" (total person) concept of health care.

Quote of the week: Thomas Edison said it best in 1880, *"The doctor of the future will give no medicine but will interest his patients in the care of the human frame in diet and in the cause and prevention of disease."*

Chiropractic entering mainstream

Question: It seems there is a Chiropractor or massage therapist on every main street in the country. Why have these alternative health-care providers become so popular?

Answer: A recent study published in the *Annals of Internal Medicine* defined the role of complementary and alternative medical therapies which include massage and Chiropractic as the two must widely sought treatments.

The most revealing statistic was the effectiveness of alternative forms of care on the 10 most commonly reported ailments. Alternative-care providers came out on top more often. Complementary and alternative medical therapy was considered better for back conditions, arthritis, headaches, and neck conditions. Conventional medical care was considered superior for only hypertension.

The study, which questioned a sample group of 2,055 people, identified trends and consumer perceptions of health care. The bottom-line reasons you see Chiropractors and massage therapists on every street corner is they make a substantial improvement for their patients' overall health and well being.

The summary of the study determined that consumers are increasingly using alternative care to address current ailments and improve overall health. It also stated consumers are spending their own money for Chiropractic and other forms of alternative care and are becoming more responsible for choosing which care is most appropriate for them. The trend is taking place in all parts of our society, is growing, and younger people will be driving this trend well into the future.

Medical doctors are no longer the dictators of health; they are just another team member.

Quote of the week: *"Hold yourself responsible for a higher standard than anybody else expects of you. Never excuse yourself."*—Henry Wood Beecher

Chiropractic is a mainstream healing profession

Question: I am a college student and I am considering Chiropractic as my career. My concern is whether Chiropractic has become mainstream or is just an alternative profession. My question is whether the Chiropractic profession is going to be accepted by the insurance industry in the future the same way that the medical profession is accepted?

Answer: I can tell you are a good student already. You are looking into the future and gauging your opportunity and stability on facts. Chiropractic is the largest natural healing profession in the world. We started from humbled and contentious beginnings to its current state of mainstream health-care providers. Chiropractic has improved its educational and licensing systems substantially giving it an increase in public credibility and improving its market share. The public utilizes Chiropractic largely for spinal pain syndromes and has a remarkable high patient-satisfaction rate. The greatest inroads are in the private and public health care financing systems and are increasingly viewed as an effective specialty by many in the medical field.

Much of the positive evolution of Chiropractic can be ascribed to a quarter century long research effort focused on the core Chiropractic procedure of spinal manipulation (adjustment). This effort has helped bring spinal manipulation out of the investigational category to become one of the most studied forms of conservative treatment for spinal pain.

I believe Chiropractic will be integrated into all health-care systems in the near future. Patient demand and patient satisfaction is higher now than ever. People are sick and tired of being sick and tired and Chiropractic is supplying a solution.

I hope your motivation to be a Chiropractor is not generated by money alone. I guarantee you will not survive long in a healing art such as Chiropractic if that is your priority. A great mentor taught me to serve for the sake of serving, give for the sake of giving and love for the sake of loving.

Quote of the week: *"You have reached the pinnacle of success as soon as you become uninterested in money, compliments, or publicity."*—O.A. Battista

Chiropractic is unique branch of health care

Question: Is Chiropractic alternative health care?

Answer: Chiropractic is one of the largest branches of health care in the United States. Federally licensed in every state and many foreign countries, the Doctor of Chiropractic can consult with, examine, diagnose, and treat a person and then submit a diagnosis and treatment plan to an insurance company, HMO, or PPO for possible reimbursement. Doctors of Chiropractic can testify in court as expert witnesses and their opinions can be entered into court records based on their training, experience, and expertise. Professional and amateur athletes, government agencies, corporations, other health care professionals, and virtually every group of people seek advice and/or treatment from Chiropractors. Chiropractic is a unique and mainstream aspect of health care in America.

Chiropractic, because of its non-drug and non-surgical approach with emphasis on prevention and wellness care, can be considered an established alternative to traditional medical care. However, since medical health-care professionals are increasingly working with Chiropractors in the best interests of the patient, one might consider this a complimentary, combined, or cooperative approach to treatment.

Quote of the Week: *"We are what we repeatedly do. Excellence, then is not an act, but a habit."*—Anonymous

Chiropractors learn on each other

Question: I have always wondered how Chiropractors learn to treat patients and if you can hurt someone trying to adjust them on your own?

Answer: When we are Chiropractic students we use each other as human Guinea pigs. It is definitely scary having a fellow unpracticed student attempt his or her very first adjustment on you. I personally learned how influential a proper adjustment of the spine can be after receiving one that was absolutely not appropriately administered when receiving my first student treatment. My fellow Chiropractor "wanna-be" was over zealous with his powerful thrust. It didn't help that he was over 300 pounds and leaned into it. There was a loud audible release to my dorsal spine that created immediate distress. Within two hours I developed a cough and diaphragm pain that lasted a month.

There does exist something called a bad adjustment, and personally experiencing this I learned very quickly I would never give such a treatment. Amateur adjusting copycats that feel they can copy their Chiropractors adjustments on their friends, or enemies, should heed this warning. It takes knowledge, confidence, and practice—not to mention a license to perform specific Chiropractic adjustments. I suggest leaving the Chiropractic adjusting to the professionals. Chiropractors are the only doctors that are trained to perform specific, gentle, corrective adjustments to remove vertebral subluxations of your spine, allowing the expression of life and health to be experienced to its highest potential.

Quote of the week: *"Spring is natures way of saying 'Let's party!'"*—Robin Williams

Chiropractors help our military

Question: Is it true Chiropractors were part of the medical team treating our soldiers in Iraq?

Answer: Yes is it is true Chiropractors were an essential part of the healing forces keeping our troops healthy and sharp. I have been hearing more and more reports of their courageous services from my colleagues as well as soldiers serving our country.

The truth is Chiropractors have been part of our military for many years. Recently a bill was passed for implementing $18 million in funding for Chiropractic benefits for active-duty military personnel in 2004. This is an increase of $6 million over what was requested in the prior year. This bill (HR 1588) was approved by the Congressional Armed Services Committee. In their statement, they indicated, "High quality health care is essential for attracting and preserving the best qualified personnel for military services."

There was a time, not so long ago, that if we were successful in getting a Chiropractic provision into a congressional bill, it had to be done quickly and in the dead of night. Now proponents of legislation are using Chiropractic as one of their selling points.

I respect and honor all the healing practitioners that perform service for our armed forces abroad and at home. They are among many of the unsung heroes of our country. I am proud to know that our government is acknowledging the multi-disciplinary approach to health care for military personnel. Our country does stand for freedom and especially freedom of choice when it comes to how we choose our health care. I only hope that the position our government has taken with the military will transfer over to our Medicare and major medical systems, which are diminishing coverage rather than increasing it.

Quote of the week: *"Quality is never an accident; it is the result of high intention, sincere effort, intelligent direction, and skillful execution: it represents the wide choice of many directions."*—Willa A. Foster

Conditioning, stretching prevent sports injuries

Question: Every basketball season my son pulls a hamstring in one of the first games. What can he do to prevent early season injuries?

Answer: Preparation and conditioning reduce injuries early in the athletic season and throughout the lifetime of a young or developed athlete.

Always prepare your cardiovascular system. Even young athletes need to have endurance and lung power. Always build your endurance on a steady gradient. You may want to start 2 to 3 months prior to your sporting season, unless you cross train year round. Walking, treadmill, biking and swimming develop increased lung capacity.

Stretching all the musculoskeletal system (muscles, ligaments, and joints) increases full ranges of motion and elongates soft tissue. Early preparation prevents sprain/strain injuries when sudden extreme jolts or traumas occur.

Know your sport and know which muscles have more demand for utilization. For example tennis and basketball require a high degree of foot pivoting so stretch the ankles and knees by isolating the calf, hamstring, quadriceps and anterior leg muscles. Team coaches, trainers or Chiropractors are great places to start for information and guidance.

Most young athletes don't need to over tax their joints with excessive heavy weight lifting. Before the age of 18 most secondary growth centers are not fully established making joints prone to permanent injuries especially with repetitive heavy weight training.

Use common sense and don't utilize a joint or muscles if it gives you persistent pain or restriction. Consult a sports injury specialist such as a Chiropractor.

Quote of the week: *"Everything we live through leaves some mark on us."*—Eugene Ionesco

Correction of leg length helps the spine

Question: Does the equal length of my legs play a role in the balance of my spine?

Answer: Most Chiropractors utilize a leg check to start their evaluation of your postural biomechanics. The leg length can reveal imbalances in many structures from the head to the feet. One of the diagnostic steps in determining if an appropriate correction was made during your treatment is to measure as to whether the legs that were uneven initially corrected to an even length. Many factors play a role in this type of diagnostic approach.

A congenital leg-length deficiency can stem from multiple causes. Polio or infections such as Leg Calf-Perthes Disease, which occur at birth, can affect growth plates on one side creating a lack of development in the hip or leg bones resulting in a congenital short leg. A severe trauma to the hips spine or legs can permanently change leg length through damage to tissues surrounding the lower torso joints. A post-surgical prosthesis mending a bone or damaged joint can also result in a leg-length deficiency. A true leg-length deficiency should be measured on X-ray as well as using two fixed positions on the hip and ankle.

A research paper conducted by Kakushima, M, et al. published in *Spine* magazine stated that patients who have leg-length discrepancy due to disorders in the lower extremities are at a greater risk of developing disabling spinal disorders due to exaggerated degenerative change. Therefore, treatment for leg-length discrepancy may be helpful in preventing degenerative spinal changes.

Treatment of permanent deficiencies may be the application of a lift or an orthotic in the shoe. In extreme cases the shoe may be built up on the outside. Should you have back pain, a visit to your Chiropractor would help determine the solution.

Quote of the week: *"It is our choices…that show what we truly are, far more than our abilities."*—J.K. Rowling

Costs spiral out of control

Question: My health-care costs for my family almost doubled last year. It is next to impossible to budget this into our lives even with two decent incomes. Even with the increase I have a deductible and co-pays. My family's health is a priority but what can I do to minimize the costs?

Answer: Spending on health care grew seven times faster than the overall economy last year, an unsustainable pace. Next year will only be worse because when you go to a doctor or even fill a prescription you may have the costs taken directly out of your paychecks to cover the health insurance. I consider this the "trickling down effect."

Employers feel the squeeze from the medical insurance hike rates and they attempt to redistribute the increased financial liability throughout their business. It could mean increases in the costs of their products or decreased benefits to their employees. An employer has to keep his or her business afloat based on economical changes. Unfortunately employees have to share the equivalent shock wave of the effect. Health insurance is the primary concern for all Americans presently. Health-care costs are out of control.

Managed-care plans attempted to offer lower co-payments and coverage of preventive services and prescription plans but had many shortcomings. They did too much managing and not enough caring. You had limited physicians and lots of overcrowding along with long waits and poor quality care. The results of this were to give more choices but increase to double-digit hikes in insurance premiums.

The simple fact is that society needs to control health-care spending. Health-care costs are complex, and it is better that patients and their doctors consider treatment costs than be bound by intrusive administrative rules. There are alternative opportunities to economize without major sacrifices. Discuss all possibilities with your insurance company and your doctors as well as speak to your political representatives to voice your views. This is America and we have a voice about freedoms and the way we receive health care.

Quote of the week: *"Do noble things, do not dream them all day."*—Charles Kinglsey

Cranial symmetry essential in infants

Question: My child was born with cranial imbalances and his head was much larger on the back of his skull on one side. Is it true there are Chiropractic techniques that can help this condition?

Answer: You described a condition in the skull called sub-occipital bulge. There is commonly a facial asymmetry associated with the condition also. The condition is due to fetal positioning prior to birth, or it can be as the infant moves through the birth canal, or during the delivery itself. The skull bones are soft and pliable on the fetus. An amazing phenomenon occurs as the large skull moves through the narrow birth canal. The two parietal bones (two bones creating the midline of the skull) overlap and then retract back into position, similar to a rebound of a sponge that was squeezed out of shape and then returned to its original shape. The inability for this to occur can influence cranial shaping. Forceps and vacuum suction devices used in delivery can also influence cranial asymmetries. Excessive strain on the occipital bones (bones in the back of your head) during any phase of birth can strain these bones leading to a variety of symptoms for the newborn including; torticollis, fever, loss of appetite, central nervous system disorders, swelling of one side of the facial soft tissues, asymmetrical development of the skull, hips, and pain sensitivity to light touch.

Chiropractic is very effective in these conditions. Two studies done on these syndromes, one in 1987 and one in 1992, treated more than 600 babies for occipital strain. The bottom line results were that most of the patients returned to normal between one to three visits. The most common irritation found in the babies was an atlas (first cervical vertebra) fixation. An adjustment of this vertebra, which anatomically lies just underneath the occiput, frees neurological flow to many cranial structures and tissues. The brain stem extends beyond the skull and is protected by the first two cervical vertebrae. This may explain why so many of the symptoms immediately rectify themselves once pressure is released and normal nerve supply restored.

Quote of the week: *"Nobody grows old merely by living a number of years. People grow old by deserting their ideals."*—Samuel Ullman

Discuss self-destructive habits with physician

Question: I am concerned about my husband's self-destructive health habits. He smokes cigarettes all day and eats everything in sight. He is overweight and his breathing is labored. My question is why his doctors don't talk to him and tell him the danger he is in?

Answer: Half the deaths in the United States are due to self-destructive behaviors, like your husband's, including smoking and overeating.

About 1.3 million people die each year from conditions that could have been prevented or delayed by healthier habits.

I don't know why your husband's doctors don't discuss his health habits. A study at Case Western Reserve University studied patient satisfaction in discussing behavioral issues.

Only 48 percent of physicians discussed behavioral issues during office visits. Discussing diet, exercise, alcohol, drug use and prevention of sexually transmitted diseases does not put off most physicians.

The study indicated patient satisfaction was much higher for those patients whose doctors did discuss behavioral concerns.

I believe healing comes from inside out. All patients are inevitably responsible for their own decisions on their health behaviors. It is absolutely the treating doctor's responsibility to alert and inform their patients of their potential self-damaging behaviors. The doctor can offer advice for counseling or alternatives to avoid the self-defeating actions.

Your husband may need a grater motivational boost to make his decision to stop his self-destruction. Lead through example of your own integrity and keep improving yourself. Leave alternatives out for him to see or read. Talk to his physicians and request they speak to him about these behaviors.

Quote of the week: *"The seasons do not push one another; neither do clouds race the wind across the sky. All things happen in their own good time."*—Dan Millman

Doctor visits cause anxiety

Question: Whenever I go to the doctor, and it can be any type of doctor, my blood pressure goes sky high. Is there a real condition that makes people over excited every time they go to a doctor?

Answer: The term used to describe your response to doctor visits is 'white coat syndrome' and it truly is categorized as a medical condition. The condition is experienced by the patient's anxiety over being examined or treated by a doctor. It originally got its label because medical doctors whom wore white traditional lab coats reported the majority of cases. The white coats became such a stigmatism due to the pre-eminent danger the doctor might incur or the bad news he may inform the patient of that many doctors and hospitals eliminated the traditional white coat.

Patients with this condition report symptoms of hypertension, headaches, dizziness and stomach distress when confronted with a trip to the doctor. A study in Italy was evenly divided as to the opinion of whether the symptoms warranted treatment. Some physicians suggested that patients exercise, while others felt the condition was a basic anxiety reaction. All agreed that if the hypertension response was extremely high or consistent it should be treated.

The condition is rarely complicated or dangerous but should be attended to. We rarely see this type of patient in our Chiropractic office. Convexly, I see patients that express that their symptoms existed until they came in to our office and mysteriously disappeared.

I believe that if this is a consistently reoccurring problem that psychological support should be sought. A prior disturbing experience with a doctor as a youth could subliminally be re-entering the mind and disturb the present time conscious physiological state of being. Without any recognition of the prior experience, your body can react to even the thought of this unpleasant time. It is important to handle this fear or reaction now, for if you require the emergency service of a doctor in the future it could complicate the condition.

Quote of the week: *"They paved paradise and put up a parking lot."*—Joni Mitchell

Chiropractic helps earaches in children

Question: My son has had earaches since he was a year old. He is now five and the earaches continue even after different series of anti-biotic treatments and tubes. Is there anything that a Chiropractor can do to help?

Answer: As a Chiropractor that focuses on pediatric conditions, I would rate earaches as one of the top five reasons that parents bring their children in to see us for treatment.

Earaches are commonly treated with anti-biotics in the medical field. A growing concern over the over-utilization and questionable effectiveness of anti-biotic use for a child's ear infection is evident. Many physicians in all the healing arts are taking precautions before writing or suggesting prescriptions for anti-biotics. The modern bacterial strains that cause ear infections are becoming more resistant to the anti-biotics. More physicians are taking cultures proper to prescribing anti-biotics, intending to get a specific antibiotic for a specific strain.

It is true that even bacterial-induced ear infections can resolve on their own. Our protocol in Chiropractic is to monitor any fevers or symptoms while administrating specific adjustments to the spine that indirectly assist the nervous system in stimulating the immune system. Additional lymphatic drainage and cranial balancing will align structures around the ear to assure proper drainage of pressure caused by congestion.

The Eustachian tubes and their position within the ear play an important role in fluid drainage from the ear. The tube angle in a young child is more horizontal than it is vertical. Because of this tube angle fluid has a tendency to remain stationary longer than when the anatomy matures to a greater vertical angle. Understanding this basic maturation process is somewhat comforting to a parent that feels their child's condition is helpless or they may need tubes pre-maturely. Each child is genetically unique in this maturation process. A possible cause of some children's tendency towards ear conditions may be this genetic predisposition.

Chiropractic has excellent success with both acute and chronic earache conditions in children. It is the responsibility of your Chiropractor to discuss every alternative and option in making a treatment choice for your child. A conservative, non-invasive drugless approach, with safety in mind first, makes the most sense.

Quote of the week: *"Life shrinks or expands in proportion to your courage."*—Barbara Winter

Cold weather can affect joints

Question: Ever since it got cold out my joints and muscles have gotten sore. Does the cold weather affect the joints and muscles and does warming them up make them feel better?

Answer: This has been a long cold winter already and yes the cold weather can affect the joints and muscles. Athletes warm up before performing their athletic events in order to stretch and prepare the muscles and joints for movement. It is called a warm up because heat allows for expansion of muscle tissue and prepares the muscles, which move joints, to move more freely and without interruption. A cold muscle maintains toxins and is more rigid. Muscles are intended to be smooth and elastic. The cold muscle does not expand as easily as the warmed up muscle. A sudden movement of a cold muscle can jerk or tear the tendons (the ends of the muscle) because it was not stretched or warmed up. Small micro tears as well as large tears in the tendons or anywhere along a muscle will cause an inflammatory reaction. Fluid is drawn to and accumulated at the site of the tear as a healing mechanism. This fluid accumulation is what interferes with joint function and may cause pain and stiffness. Whether you are an athlete or a non-athlete, a cold muscle that is taxed for activity prior to appropriate preparation is asking for trouble especially in the cold weather. When your body temperature is down it takes even more of a warm up to prepare muscles and joints.

To combat the achy muscle/joint winter syndrome I suggest always dressing warm. Drink plenty of fluids, both warm and cold, especially water. Do moderate stretching of every joint after your morning shower. Yoga is an excellent form of daily preparation. Anti-oxidants such as Vitamin C and Vitamin E along with MSM, glucosamine sulfate and/or chondroiton sulfate have been documented to reduce joint aches. Discuss these alternatives with your medical physician or Chiropractor

Your doctor should review persistent joint or muscle ache that progresses or is very intense. Chiropractors are an excellent source of knowledge and may have procedures that can help your condition.

Quote of the week: *"The difference between ordinary and extraordinary is that little extra."*—Anonymous

Embrace wellness for the New Year

Question: What would you consider the healthiest New Year's resolution?
Answer: I consider family wellness care with Chiropractic treatments on a regular basis the healthiest resolution you and your family could make. There is nothing more important than your health and the health of your loved ones. When priorities take precedence in a series of qualifying decisions in life, the greatest priority is your health. There is no greater level of expression of "quality of life" than feeling healthy. If you have ever suffered with low-back pain, neck pain, headaches or just fatigue, it most likely ruined your holiday or the enjoyable time you could have had.

Neither money, toys, nor vacations can compensate for well being. You can not enjoy the money, vacation or toys when your mind and body aren't functioning properly. He who has the most toys does not necessarily win, especially if you die early.

Chiropractors provide a natural painless holistic approach to health-care maintenance. The nervous system controls the functions of all your cells, tissues and organs. Chiropractors detect and correct irritations to your nervous system called vertebral subluxations. Any form of stress, whether it is emotional, chemical, physical, family, job, relationships, etc., can contribute to an adverse response in your nervous system (the vertebral subluxation). Chiropractic is positioned as the only health-care profession that focuses on the absolute cause of neurological dysfunction. By gently adjusting the vertebrae, Chiropractors release the imbalances in the nervous system caused by the overabundance of stress.

Maintenance of your spine to balance your nervous system should be a priority for any family concerned about their quality of life and health.

Intelligent families educate themselves and shift responsibilities to make time to get to their Chiropractic appointments. The minimal amount of sacrifice and cost it takes to maintain your health is monumentally exceeded by the benefits reaped in having a healthy family.

I may seem extreme in my advice for your New Year's resolution, because after 22 years of practice I can tell you Chiropractic treated families are happier and healthier.

Quote of the week: *"People can alter their lives by altering their attitudes."*—William James

Epidural injections rarely work

Question: I have had low-back pain with sciatica for six months. I tried Chiropractic, physical therapy and oral medications and nothing has helped. My pain-management doctor suggested a series of three epidural injections and I really thought this should kill the pain. They didn't work either. Why wouldn't even epidural injections work to help my pain?

Answer: Your question is one I hear every day. Most physicians that utilize epidural injections will communicate to their patients that the anti-inflammatory and painkiller agents will only sustain temporary relief. My clinical experience with consulting more than 1,000 different patients whom received these injections is that they rarely reduce pain and rarely remove any symptoms of low-back pain or sciatica.

A study that was published in *The New England Journal of Medicine* was titled "Epidural Injections: No Significant Benefit for Sciatica." This article in June of 1999 concluded that epidural-corticosteriod injections commonly used for low-back pain and sciatica had not established any efficacy. The article claimed that some patients received short-term pain relief but it did not reduce the need for surgery.

Patients such as you, with excruciating low-back pain and sciatica that get no relief have had very few options in the past. Today there are more options. Chiropractic has evolved to have more scientific and specific treatments for low-back pain. Acupuncture has been a great source of pain relief for many patients. Deep myofacial massage can be very effective to reduce muscle spasms. The Beachwood Low Back Rehab Center offers a non-invasive treatment for low-back conditions called VAX-D therapy, which is 75-percent successful. You can learn more about this treatment and others at Web site www.beachwoodlowback.com.

Quote of the week: *"Many hands and hearts and minds generally contribute to anyone's notable achievements."*—Walt Disney

Examine what your insurance plan will, won't cover

Question: I pay a lot of money for my health insurance and purchased it because it advertised that it covered alternative healthcare such as massage and acupuncture. I finally went to use my insurance and found out that this is not true at all? Why are insurance companies allowed to false advertise like this?

Answer: Unfortunately we hear this complaint from many of our patients on a daily basis. Deceptive advertising to get your expensive contract seems to be an industry standard. There is one particular company that lures its susceptible clients with loud declarations of coverage for all alternative treatments because they care. Their policies have small print and exceptions that read quite the opposite to their declarations. Sure, if you get a referral from your primary physician and pay out of network slightly less than the actual cost of the treatment you can go.

Massage therapists and acupuncturists have been very concerned with these faux policies and the ones I know just laugh when they hear that insurance will cover their services. They relay to me that they get calls daily by potential ailing patients who believe they have coverage and specifically bought the insurance just so they could get these alternative treatments.

There are dozens of alternative health-care treatments available, almost as many as the number of candidates in the California gubernatorial race.

If the insurance companies are going to continue to pronounce their new liberal progressive support of the alternative health-care movement then why don't they just cover all forms of alternative care. Lets start with massage, acupuncture, light therapy, color therapy, aroma therapy, isolation tanks, meditation, yoga, chanting, pyramid power, and lets not forget alien worship. It won't be long before insurance companies become our best friends, NOT! For now, you will continue to pay deductibles higher than your mortgage payments and co-pays larger than car payments.

Good luck at changing the system. Financially supported insurance lobbyist have such a stronghold on lawmakers it will take crowbars to separate them.

My advice is to search the web for small insurance groups that support alternative healthcare at an affordable rate. Read your policies and ask your insurance agent to review the exact details of how your health-care coverage works. It is risky, but many people are choosing no insurance coverage or just can't afford it.

Quote of the week: *"Once in a while it really strikes people that they don't have to live in the way they have been told to."*—Alan Keightly

Follow Mother Theresa's lead

Question: Many patients come in daily, disgusted with the state of human relations and their interactions with people on a daily basis. They have progressively been sharing with me that people are becoming mean and inconsiderate. They ask if I know why?

Answer: I would like to attend to this unfortunate but often asked question with a quote from Mother Theresa, "God does not command that we do great things, only little things with great love."

When we get overwhelmed with negative experiences we sometimes are consumed by negative thoughts. It takes great discipline to remove the onslaught of a series of unpleasant episodes. Forgiveness is essential and changing your perspective is even more beneficial. It is essential to discipline ourselves to focus on the "little things." The "things" that are good and positive. The general overwhelming state of affairs can appear grim at times but you can erase the displeasure by concentrating on the small stuff such as loved ones in your life. In any situation I first ask myself if my children's lives are endangered by the actions at hand. Second, I determine if my health or welfare is endangered. If no danger or health risk exists then it is just small and insignificant to me. You will find that 90 percent of the so-called "bad stuff" truly is insignificant.

Develop a "Teflon" attitude to verbal abuse and abhorrent behaviors of others. Lead through example. Reacting with anger, formulating retaliation or acting irreverently only hardens a bad situation. According to some patients there are plenty of "bad situations" to practice being "Teflon" to.

Raise your standards and take control of yourself. Life is an ongoing learning experience. By meeting the challenge and overcoming adversity you will become empowered. Choose to be more caring and compassionate. You will be more powerful and happier in the end.

Foot injuries should be taken seriously

Question: My son recently stubbed his toes into the dining room table. I didn't know whether he broke his toes or how to treat him. What would you recommend?

Answer: Home injuries with the feet should always be taken seriously. The criteria to determine if emergency treatment is needed includes; extreme distortion of the joint from its normal position, excessive swelling, discoloration, pain and/or referred pain. You may still have a fracture without these symptoms or only a few of them. As a parent, your biggest concern is that a growth plate hasn't been damaged. Growth plates at the end of bones are where the bone develops with its nutritional supply. A distortion in the endplate could produce improper development as your child grows, and permanent changes.

In a trauma with any joint, ice should be administered immediately along with visual inspection. The degree of pain is usually an accurate measurement of the degree of the injury. If there is any doubt that there may be a fracture, diagnostic X-rays should be taken to determine their presence. If a fracture is ruled out then the condition is commonly an injury to the supporting ligaments, and muscles around the feet, toes and ankle. This is considered a sprain/strain trauma and many times can involve more radical symptoms than a fracture. It should be immobilized and rested initially. Restoring motion back to the joint as soon as possible after the acute phase of healing is essential to minimize scar formation which may lead to future adhesions that restrict motion.

Adjustments of extremities after a trauma, such as a jammed toe or other digit, can restore motion and enhance the healing process.

Quote of the week: *"The price of greatness is responsibility."*—Winston Churchill

Generosity may lead to longevity of life

Question: I volunteer at the hospital and find that when I give my time to others I feel better. Is it true that when you give of yourself it helps your overall health?

Answer: Generosity of spirit absolutely yields emotional and physical healing benefits. Social contact improves health and promotes longer life. Ocean County has a very large population of retired seniors that can make an extraordinary impact on the health and well being of the community with donated social volunteering. I believe true givers give without the expectation of being rewarded, however the rewards of improved health and longevity are worth the small sacrifice for voluntary service.

A study by psychologist Stephanie Brown at the University of Michigan studied 423 couples and set a baseline by asking the individuals if they had given or received more emotional and practical help in the past year. Five years later the study revealed that those who said they'd helped others were half as likely to have died than the receivers.

The "Helpers High" as coined by psychologist Robert Cialdini of Arizona State University describes the euphoria frequent givers experience. These good feelings may lower the output of stress hormones, which improves cardiovascular health and strengthens the immune system.

Living by the old adage "it's more blessed to give than receive" now carries a potent message especially for the elderly. Giving generously and regularly lengthens your life span and improves your health.

Quote of the week: *"Blessed are those who can give without remembering and take without forgetting."*—Elizabeth Bibesco

Good patients keep their appointments

Question: What is the most difficult or frustrating part of being a Chiropractor when it comes to patient-doctor relations?

Answer: Missed appointments ranks up there as a top frustration for me as a Chiropractor trying to give my patients the best quality care possible. Specific schedules are given to specific patients for specific conditions. There are not any two conditions that are identical. Our bodies develop patterns of adaptation to our conditions which affect our entire physical, emotional and chemical being. When a patient starts their treatment it is imperative to get an opportunity to determine how they respond to treatment. There are protocols to diagnose and treat based on response. When the patient misses appointments it is difficult to manage their patterns of their condition. Most conditions take time to develop and also take time to heal. Many patients claim it was the last task or movement that created their pain or symptom when in reality it is the final reaction of a series of events or patterns that led up to the one that gave them the symptom. Patients that want a quick fix of their problem might as well take a drug and mask the condition. In Chiropractic care our goal is to find the cause and correct it. Sometimes it only takes a few treatments and sometimes it may take a year. In either case, the doctor-patient relationship is very important and having the respect and confidence in your Chiropractor will only benefit you. Missing scheduled appointments, especially without notification is disrespectful and interferes with appropriate care.

In the same vein of respect for the patient, a doctor should not make their patient wait if they are scheduled at a specific time. Everyone seems to have an agenda these days and time is precious. Making a patient wait for excessive time beyond their appointment is also disrespectful.

I have found that patients that keep appointments throughout care get better quicker and maintain their health at a higher potential.

Quote of the week: *"When in doubt, tell the truth."* Mark Twain

Healing has much to do with doctor's intent

Question: I have been a patient of a few different Chiropractors and I find that even though they give similar treatments only one really makes me feel great. Why does this occur?

Answer: Chiropractic has evolved over the last 100 years to utilize many different means, yet to satisfy the same ends. The Chiropractor's primary goal is to remove interference from the nervous system to allow the body to express itself as close to 100 percent as possible. Your body always does the healing, not the doctor. That's right, your body has the ability to heal itself. As human beings we tend to challenge our bodies by exposing it to various undue stress. Overtaxing stress can come from a physical, mental or chemical source. It can come from family, friends, jobs or simple life itself. We adapt to change daily, even second to second. Interruption of our nervous system that controls all other systems including our immune system, endocrine system (hormone balance), digestive system etc., alters the perfection of function in our body. Chiropractors work with the protective coverings of the nervous system the skull, spinal column, pelvis and extremities along with their surrounding connective tissues, muscles, ligaments and cartilage to restore homeostasis.

Since the final goal, neurological balance, hasn't changed nor the correction of neurological dysfunction (vertebral subluxations) then the techniques must be the new variable. Chiropractic has a multitude of techniques to accomplish corrections. I cannot name all of them but here are a few of the most common ones:

Activator, the hand-held spring device that varies in depth and force;

<u>Sacro-Occipital Technique (SOT)</u>, a technique of balancing the upper and lower ends of the spine utilizing pelvic blocking, cranial balancing, and light adjusting;

<u>Pierce, Diversified and Gonstead</u>, hands on techniques that specifically correct subluxations based on postural distortions and diagnostic procedures; and

<u>Upper cervical/toggle techniques</u>, specific adjustments using quick reflex adjusting of the upper cervical region.

There are many more and all work.

The answer to your question regarding why two different Chiropractors using the same techniques get different results is theoretically one of these reasons. You are more receptive to the Chiropractor giving the positive result or the Chiropractor giving the negative result may not have appropriate intent. Intention and focus of any type of doctor while administering treatment is the key element to success with his or her patient. A friend of mine once said the majority of people are touched in society for only two reasons, to be made love to or to be harmed. When a patient is touched by his or her Chiropractor, that doctor should be focusing on only the benefit and correction that patient will receive. The patient should have total confidence in the Chiropractor that he or she will detect and correct their vertebral subluxations to the best of their ability with their best intention. When the giver and receiver are in harmony healing occurs. Many times, it is not so much the technique used by Chiropractors but their intent. When you and your Chiropractor have this relationship it is a great idea to stick with them.

Quote of the week: *"Vitality shows not only in the ability to persist but in the ability to start over."*—F. Scott Fitzgerald

Healthy diet needs balance

Question: There are so many diets, authorities and books telling us different ways to eat. I am confused about what is the best way to eat to stay healthy. What is your opinion on the guidelines to a healthy diet?

Answer: There are definite methods and protocols to eating healthy. I will give you my guidelines to maintaining a healthy diet.

- Eat a balanced meal within an hour after waking. This jump-starts your blood sugar and hormones.

- Eat small, frequent meals. You will keep the fat-burning process going, never feel hungry and prevent the high and low peaks of energy. Three balanced meals and two snacks a day with no more than 5 hours between meals is recommended.

- Drink more water. Six to eight 10-ounce glasses per day are average for a 150-pound person.

- Eat more fiber. Increase fruits and vegetables. Minimize pasta, cereals, breads, rice and potatoes.

- Eat less fat in the form of fried greasy foods. Supplement with omega three fatty acids (including flaxseed oil or fish oils).

Don't worry so much. If you blow your diet, you can start again at your next meal. The idea is to live better, not to beat yourself up for making mistakes. We all learn this process the hard way.

Don't drink your calories. You can gain excess weight from high caloric drinks and ruin all your good work with a solid diet.

Stay adjusted. Chiropractors help maintain a healthy functioning nervous system which directly influences the balance of your digestive system.

Quote of the week: *"Courage is the capacity to confront what can be imagined."*—Leo Roster

Healthy home environment prevents winter colds

Question: Is it possible that I am getting sick due to the heater in my house? Since I turned on the system my nose runs and I feel terrible. Can your home environment cause illness?

Answer: Your home environment absolutely can contribute to a weakened immune system leading to illness. The winter season has an extreme influence on our internal home environments. Closed windows trap airborne viruses, bacteria and mold. When improper circulation of air is present these germs can become static and multiply. Repetitive cleaning of potential sources of the germs is helpful but it may only scratch the surface of a serious exposure to the cause of the problem. Some tips for winter household health maintenance include:

1. Clean all vents, ductwork, chimneys and baseboard elements.

2. Remove dust and pollen accumulated on windows, paddle fans, ceilings, walls and floors.

3. Have your house checked for mold if there has been a history of water leaks prior in the year. If you smell a mold odor or suspect mold in your vents call a professional to analyze your heating, air and ventilation systems.

4. Air purifiers are an exceptional way to collect airborne germs and allergens on a daily basis.

5. Check to maintain proper humidity levels in your home. A dry environment may create dry mucous membranes in the sinuses and throat contributing to potential irritation or infection.

6. Be aware of the materials used to build your home and make sure toxic materials, such as asbestos, are removed.

Persistent conditions and illness should not be left untreated. Chiropractors are trained professionals in the health field that may help your immune system recover by balancing your nervous system.

Quote of the week: *"Looking back, we see with great clarity, and what once appeared as difficulties now reveal themselves as blessings."*—Dan Millman

Hiatal hernias mimic heart attacks

Question: I consulted several doctors about indigestion high in my stomach that causes chest pain. Some felt it was a hiatal hernia. What can be done naturally to help this condition?

Answer: A hiatal hernia is the spilling of gas or gastric tissue upward through an opening in your diaphragm. In severe cases surgery may be required to pull the tissue back to its original position. Most cases, similar to what you describe in your condition, are the pressure of gastric gas moving into the space between your diaphragm muscle, located under your ribs, and your stomach. As you ascend and descend your ribs through normal phases of respiration a pressure and pain can occur due to this stomach gas. The pressure and pain can radiate throughout your chest and into your back. The pain can be so severe in the left chest wall many people feel like they are having a heart attack.

Treatment on a conservative basis can consist of dealing with the cause of the condition, the gas. The gas is commonly caused by undigested food in the stomach. Many people hold their stress in their stomachs or eat while on the move, or just eat very poorly. A combination of these situations can lead to an overabundance of gas leading to pressure in the diaphragm due to hiatal hernia. Proper diet and avoiding gassy foods is helpful. Eating slowly and chewing your food well is important. Persistent hiatal hernias that are not in need of medical attention may be helped with Chiropractic treatment. There are gentle procedures to help release the gas causing pressure on the diaphragm. Adjustments can reduce pressure in the chest and spine related to a hiatal hernia.

Quote of the week: *"Cherish your visions and your dreams as they are the children of your soul; the blueprints of your ultimate achievements."*—Napoleon Hill

High heels pose a potential hazard

Question: I wear high heels and have been told they are bad for my feet and back. I prefer the way I look with heels. Is it bad to wear high heels?

Answer: Many women patients of ours have decided to wear more comfortable shoes for daily business and at home use. Besides feeling safer, they wear them because it's healthier.

High heels force an unnatural posture upon the foot and low back. High heels shorten the muscles of the calves and compromise this muscle group with extended wear. These types of footwear put all the weight forward on the balls of the feet (metatarsals), which is naturally intended to be redistributed equally across the entire foot.

I am always concerned about long term high heel utilization when considering the Chiropractic model of spinal balance. High heels shove the pelvis forward stressing the lower back, forcing it into an unnatural, dangerously misaligned curve. It is very common to observe chronic low pack pain as a symptom of women wearing high heels.

Estimations indicate that the average American takes over 10,000 steps each day. That is more than 3.5 million steps each year. Compromising your feet, legs, pelvis and low back for glamour is a personal decision that should be reconsidered.

Quote of the week: *"You cannot shake hands with a closed fist."*—Golda Meir

Holiday stress-reduction tips

Follow tips to reduce stress of holiday season

During the holiday season, we can allow many situations and circumstances to create extra stress in our lives. During the next few weeks, I will share some ways to reduce the stress of the season. First, a list of things to do:

- **Soothe with food:** Eat several mini-meals between meals of natural carbohydrates. They elevate mood-regulating brain chemical, serotonin, which exerts a calming effect on the entire body.

- **Ask three questions:** Is this important? Is my reaction appropriate? Is this situation changeable? Take action to change it.

- **Exercise:** Physical activity reduces anxiety and depression. Aerobic exercise is best but choose and exercise that you enjoy.

- **Check your perspective:** Do only the tasks that would have serious consequences if left undone. Will you die if you don't do the laundry?

- **Skip some routine chores:** Take at least a half-hour daily to do something you enjoy to recharge yourself.

- **Take a mini-breather:** Belly breathe throughout the day periodically. It keeps oxygen going to your brain and slows you down in anxious moments.

- **Look at the light side:** A good laugh relaxes muscles, lowers blood pressure and suppresses stress-related hormones.

- **Reduce caffeine:** Caffeine is a stimulant that runs up the nervous system and makes you more susceptible to stress. A good replacement is green tea.

- **Take a time out:** An overloaded schedule causes anxiety. Schedule a half-hour of nothing in a workday. If emergencies or calls come in, you have extra time.

- **Say a little prayer:** Prayer reduces stress hormones and balances emotions. It gives you inner calm and can help "heal thyself."

- **Make a list of likes and dislikes:** List as a family what parts of the holiday each likes and dislikes. Eliminate as many dislikes as possible.

- **Shop year round:** Buy gifts throughout the year rather than wait until the last minute. Start baking and cooking earlier for those items that will stay fresh.

Next week: The list continues.

Tips help reduce holiday stress

I previously offered some suggestions to combat the propensity of allowing many situations and circumstances to create extra stress in our lives. Here are some ideas to keep things from getting too intense during this season (and it wouldn't be a bad idea to incorporate some of these ideas when making New Year's resolutions):

Divide the chores: Divide the family into responsibilities so no one person totes the load.

Let family and friends know what you are doing: It's OK to not send cards, make fruitcakes, or even give gifts. Let people know your intentions and, to your surprise, it will be fine. In fact, they will envy you.

Compromise on the excess of activities: Reduce your traditional activities based on your family's enjoyment level. Don't cram so much into a short time; spontaneity is a beautiful thing.

Consider your origins and traditions: Rehash with your family how your personal traditions came about. Focus on love and spirit. Pass on the true meaning of the holidays.

Celebrate Christmas for the kids: Be a kid yourself. Stop and look at your kid's letters to Santa, write one yourself. If no kids, go to a hospital or a shelter and be around them. They are spiritual and clear.

Remember your pets and the animals: Spend time with your pets, contribute time to a shelter, or just contemplate our coexistence with the animal kingdom.

Celebrate Mother Earth: Acknowledge the seasonal changes honoring the earth and protecting our environment.

Give anonymously: Give to your church or neighbor to help a struggling human being. Give a hug if that's all you can afford.

Have a silent night: Extended times of quiet allow us to become spiritually in tune and contemplate our lives without distraction.

Spend time with the elderly: The wisdom of the past and the view from before is imperative for the youth of families to maintain tradition, custom, and respect.

Cut down on your Christmas card list: Reduce your time. Don't send to people you haven't heard from or dealt with for extended time.

Cut back the number of gifts to kids: Kids get the wrong impression of what Christmas is about. Teach lessons in value. Give less, pay more.

Teach your kids to give: Attempt to take kids away from the self-centered materialistic world we live in.

Less is more: It is the little things that count—gestures of kindness, mints on the pillow, listening and loving.

Create a countdown to Christmas: Make a timeline for each day as to what will be done on each day leading to Christmas.

Stop and smell the flowers: Make it a point to live life's natural splendors. Smell the morning air, watch a sunrise, watch a sunset, look at the stars, and go to the ocean or into the woods. Use your senses of smell, taste, feel, listen and see. Visualize, dream, and be happy.

Get adjusted: See your Chiropractor frequently during stressful times to maximize your health and well being!

Keep stress of holidays at bay

In the past couple of weeks, I've given you some things to reduce the stress of the holiday season. Today, I'll talk about things NOT to do to achieve the same end:

1. **Avoid the media.** Stop watching television, ads, magazines, radio and billboards. They create an unrealistic vision of what holidays should be.

2. **Don't miss meals**. Low blood sugar causes fatigue and disorientation, leading to stress and illness.

3. **Don't drive distracted**. More injuries and accidents occur during holidays than any other time of year. Focus on the road and watch out for road rage.

4. **Don't put yourself in debt**. Buy within your budget. It isn't the size of the gift, it's the heartfelt thought that goes into it.

5. **Don't buy useless gifts**. It is now the trend to purchase investments as gifts, especially for children and teens, bonds, college savings, education, and personal growth gifts.

6. **Don't exhaust yourself.** Exhaustion makes our bodies run down and susceptible to colds and flu. Take increased amounts of Vitamin C, Echinacea and drink lots of water. Most importantly, see your Chiropractor and stay in adjustment.

7. **Don't invite guests you don't like.** Don't make your home a bed and breakfast for people you don't want there, even if they are former friends or family. It's your family's holiday.

8. **Don't let guilt spoil your holiday.** Jealousy or pressure from family or environment can create feelings of guilt. Don't buy into it. Those feeling belong to the outside party, enjoy yourself.

9. **Don't compete with other families.** Holidays aren't about who spent more or how many or whose is larger. It's about the love and spirit of sharing and caring.

10. **Don't give goods—give services.** Gift certificates for movies, dinner, massages, Chiropractic exams, etc. are non-returnable and give people and experience rather than an object.

11. **Boycott Christmas mall shopping.** Don't get caught with the throngs of other stressful holiday shoppers. Shop out of a few favorite catalogues or by mail or phone.

12. **Don't get caught in the kitchen.** Prepare foods ahead of time and enjoy your guests.

13. **Don't watch television when guests visit.** Don't be distracted by sports or Nutcracker shows. This may be the only quality time you get to spend with friends and family all year.

14. **Don't drink alcohol.** Alcohol consumption is a proven depressant. With emotions already high, alcohol can increase anxiety and depression as well as lead you to act like a fool or say something you regret.

15. **Minimize sugar intake.** Sugar for kids is equivalent to adding fire to gasoline. Kids are hyper as usual. Add sugar and they bounce off the walls. Wait one hour after meals to reduce sugar reactions if you must include it.

Hot flash on hot flashes

Question: I am going through menopause and found that every woman friend my age that I discuss it with is confused and bewildered as to how to manage the condition. What can you tell me about the natural approach to dealing with the hot flashes of menopause?

Answer: Menopause is a hot topic, no pun intended. Since the recent release of the government study showing that hormone-replacement therapy does more harm than good, there's been plenty of discussion on alternatives. The government urged women to stop using estrogen and progesterone-replacement therapies when these studies linked this treatment with various cancers. Millions of women were misled to pharmaceutical companies to believe the benefits of these drugs. The companies overstated the benefits and understated the risks to obtain massive profits.

It is time for women to question authorities on the value of their medications. It is easier to simply pop the pill, whatever it is, than to study up on diet, exercise and alternatives. There are no excuses anymore. We have a plethora of information at our fingertips. When you type in the key words "hormone-replacement therapy" during an Internet search you are shown almost 100,000 sites.

Holistic medicine, Chiropractic, and herbal remedies are finally getting the respect and attention they deserve regarding menopausal changes. Menopause is not a disease, it is a natural female progression of life.

Utilize the Internet, call a Chiropractor and gather your own knowledge to make an intelligent decision on what you will do during menopause. Be a leader and your friends will respect and appreciate you for taking the initiative.

Quote of the week: *"As I see it, every day you do one to two things: build health or produce disease in yourself."*—Adele Davis

Humans shrink in height as they get older

Question: I am in my mid-60s and I feel like I have gotten noticeably shorter. Is it true we get shorter as we get older and does your spine have something to do with it?

Answer: Your entire body is made up of almost 80-percent fluid and your discs in your spine are approximately 88-percent fluid. It is a normal progression of aging to dehydrate. As healthy tissues, normally enriched with vitamins and minerals when we are younger, start to age, they loose their healthy resiliency and get dry and more rigid. The loss of fluid in tissues in the entire body in general creates a loss in height. The spinal discs make up about one sixth of our total height. It is not unusual for each disc to loose half its fluid concentration as we reach our 60s or 70s. A loss of two to three inches is common toward the end of our life span.

A healthy lifestyle may encourage a slower rate of dehydration and loss of height. The ingestion of six to eight large 8-ounce glasses of water daily helps keep all systems, especially the spinal discs, healthier. Spinal adjustments by your Chiropractor can minimize spinal compression and misalignment, which can cause spinal disc dehydration. Staying active and stimulating movement of fluid through all your joints will reduce chances of arthritis and joint deterioration. Healthy diets that avoid excess sugars, animal fats and dense carbohydrates may reduce stress on tissues, which cause them to age quicker than normal.

Some people are genetically predestined to shrink, as they get older. In this case there is not much you can do but where lifts or heals which could be slightly uncomfortable for a man. There is a difference between shrinking due to natural disposition and leaning forward due to a degenerative spine or ailing joints. Poor posture habits can be rectified in many cases prior to permanent change. Should you notice changes in your significant other, family member or in yourself, have a Chiropractor examine you to determine if there is help in correcting your posture changes.

Quote of the week: *"Endurance pierces marble."*—Moroccan Proverb

Hyper-mobility and fixation of spinal joints are both unhealthy

Question: My Chiropractor told me my spine is unhealthy because it is too hyper-mobile. He also said it makes it difficult to adjust me. What is hyper-mobility and why would it be difficult to adjust the spine because of it?

Answer: Your Chiropractor is correct on both claims. Hyper-mobility of a spinal joint means the joint is moving beyond its normal ranges of motion and there is not a restriction at the end of its full range. Some patients, especially younger ones, naturally have excessive flexibility and hyper-mobility that is considered normal for their age and activity levels. When the mature spinal joints move past their restrictive end points abnormal wear and tear can occur to the joints themselves. When the movement is excessive muscles pull from their origin and insertion, which are usually bony, prominences naturally formed on the joints. The repetitive hyper-mobile movements upon the spinal joints can create irritation to the tendons (attachments from the muscle to bone) leading to tendonitis. Other forms of inflammation can occur around the spinal joints, including arthritis, and degeneration.

The reason it is difficult for your Chiropractor to administer an adjustment to the hyper-mobile joint is because it doesn't stay in alignment once corrected. Some successful approaches to dealing with this condition are to perform gentler low force adjustments that do not require putting the joint in motion during treatment. Also, educating the patient on how to strengthen their spine will sometimes help the muscles and joints.

Fixation of a joint is more common. This is also an unhealthy spinal condition. Restriction of motion to fibrotic adhesions, also known as scar tissue, reduces activity in the joint causing it to be stagnant. Without proper motion dead tissue from normal usage builds up, making it difficult for the body to filter out bad necrotic tissue and allow healthy minerals and vitamins to restore healing to the joints.

Chiropractic adjustments are exceptional in these cases because they allow the body to heal itself by restoring normal mobility leading to normal function.

Quote of the week: *"Do not ask people to do what you are not willing to do yourself."*—Phillip Mcgraw

Infant birth conditions respond to Chiropractic

Question: My 8-week-old baby had terrible reflux and colic and after taking more than seven different drugs. I decided to try a natural approach with my Chiropractor. The results have been phenomenal. My baby now sleeps through the night and isn't in pain after every feeding. Can you share this with your readers so they know they have options?

Answer: Thank you for sharing your successful experience in the correction of infant colic and reflux. Chiropractors have been helping infants with these and many other birth-related dysfunctions for years. Our patients are educated about the importance of a healthy nervous system for their babies from birth and throughout their lives. To many it is common sense to have their baby's spine checked immediately after childbirth while those that are uneducated or have misconceptions about why a baby's spine should be checked immediately after birth conceive it as dangerous or even repulsive. Let me clearly inform those that have doubts. The amount of pressure necessary to adjust the tiny fragile vertebrae of an infant is equivalent to the pressure you would put on your closed eyelid to press it against your eyeball. I adjust infants with my pinky finger with direct precise lines of correction. We utilize something called mirror image adjusting which means putting the area of the spine that is misaligned in the exact opposite direction than its distortion. These methods re-educate muscles tissues and nerves to come to their neutral balanced position allowing for symmetrical growth. The parent usually assists me in moving their baby and always knows exactly what procedure I will do before any treatment is performed. The treatments are gentle painless and with minimal force. Always remember the body wants to right itself from improper unhealthy positioning and with just the slightest assistance will begin to heal. Infants and children respond quickly and completely in most cases because their nervous systems haven't been exposed to an overload of stress and accumulated trauma's. Infants are very responsive to a tender healing hand with correct intention and focus.

You may ask how this has anything to do with reflux and colic. Balancing the nervous system of an infant by removing interruptions in function caused by structural misalignment (vertebral subluxations) restores nerve and blood supplies to all your organs, tissues and cells. Once restored the body will heal itself. It really isn't a mystery or a faith, it is scientific reality that we are self-healing organisms and once balanced and cared for stay healthy. In the case of infant colic and reflux there is commonly subluxations of the coccyx, occipital upper cervical, and or the 12th thoracic vertebra. Cranial bone misalignments also play a role in these conditions. Working with the parents regarding nursing, types of formula, and potential allergens is extremely helpful. We also teach our infant's parents how to perform massage on their baby's to relieve gas and irritation.

Quote of the week: *"How often could things be remedied by a word. How often is it left unspoken?"*—Norman Douglas

Jaw conditions respond well to Chiropractic

Question: I was told by my physician that I have temporomandibular disease (TMD). My jaw hurts constantly and it is driving me crazy. Nothing I have done to help it, including medications, stops the pain. Can you suggest anything?

Answer: There is hope for your TMD condition. Chiropractic may be your solution. We successfully treat TMD conditions regularly in our office.

The temporomandibular joint (TMJ) acts as a sliding joint with one bone sliding upon the surface of the other. The muscles surrounding the TMJ are called the muscles of mastication (chewing). These muscles are the strongest, most powerful muscles in your body. Chewing, biting and shearing activities controlled by these muscles requires a dramatic amount of nerve and blood supply. Damage to the jaw muscles causes the excitation of the dense nerve supply and increases pain levels higher than anywhere else in your body. Besides normal nerve supply to the jaw, there are sensitive cranial nerves in the face and jaw that can be aggravated with overuse or trauma. Conditions associated with these irritations are Bell's palsy (7th cranial nerve) and trigeminal neuralgia (5th cranial nerve).

The majority of causes of jaw pain or TMD are associated with TMJ misalignment secondary to dental conditions. The bite or your teeth due to improper shifting can wear down the surface of one or both sides of the TMJ. Many times a bite guard and/or dental surface balancing will help. Bruxing (grinding your teeth at night) is a secondary effect of stress or teeth misalignment. Over time this will wear the TMJ down also.

Many Chiropractors are trained to evaluate, diagnose and treat TMD conditions. Most corrections are gentle and are as simple as a light balancing correction to the joint itself.

Quote of the week: *"Hold yourself responsible for a higher standard than anybody else expects of you. Never excuse yourself."*—Henry Ward Beecher

Job can aggravate back pain

Question: I am trying to decide on a new job and I am concerned about having low-back pain. What jobs are safer and less potentially irritating to your low back?

Answer: No job is totally immune from causing irritation to your spine. There are multiple factors to consider when deciding on a job based on spinal safety. Your own personal body shape and existing condition are important influences, as well as the degree of training and comfort already established in that vocation.

A job should give you satisfaction as well. Being under stress for emotional or environmentally unhealthy reasons on the job also can lead to back pain.

According to a *Better Homes and Gardens* article, some of the worst jobs for a bad back include farmers, foresters, commercial fisherman, doctors (including Chiropractors), dentists and nurses.

You should note that you don't have to lift heavy objects to develop low-back pain. Sitting at a desk for a long time can potentially injure your back.

Quote of the week: *"Dwell as near as possible to the channel in which your life flows."*—Henry David Thoreau

Lifestyle changes lower blood pressure

Question: Is there a way to reduce my blood pressure without taking drugs?

Answer: This is a good question considering a recent publication indicates the former "normal" blood pressure parameter of 120/80 is now considered a slightly high blood pressure.

The Journal of the American Medical Association recently did a study on the impact of a combination of lifestyle changes on high blood pressure. The good news is that mildly elevated blood pressure can be lowered without drugs.

Dr. Lawrence Appel of John Hopkins University, who chaired the study, said, "It (lifestyle changes) may be a means to control blood pressure and a lot of heart disease and stroke without actually relying on medication."

In general the group studied were counseled on weight loss, salt reduction, and increasing exercise. They were also instructed on diet information that emphasized fruits, vegetables, and low-fat dairy products along with a reduction in unhealthy fats, red meat, sweets, and sugared beverages. All but 27 of the 800 adults in the study reduced their blood pressure enough to stop drug treatment.

Additional advice on reducing blood pressure and maintaining a healthy cardiovascular system includes supplementing fish oils called essential fatty acids that come from cold-water fish. This was the first year the Food and Drug Administration (FDA) made fish, specifically cold-water fish such as cod and salmon) an essential part of our meals at least two times weekly.

Quote of the week: *"Even if you fall on your face, you're still moving forward."*—Victor Kiam

Long-standing problems require
many adjustments

Question: I have been going to a Chiropractor to get adjustments for over a year now. I must admit I do feel better, but my question is why has it taken so long to get better and why do people need so many adjustments before they are healed?

Answer: Healing takes time. It sounds cliché, but it is the truth in all-healing processes including mental healing. Growing up in America injects the premise that healing comes from the outside in as opposed to the inside out. The general media conditioning that we have been bombarded with has subliminally seduced us into believing that health and healing are similar to fast food dining. We want it when we want it we want it now. We have lots to do and we can't wait. Unfortunately, fast food dining is neither nutritious nor appropriate for proper digestion nor is expecting your health to come for a magic pill, miracle ointment or instantaneously.

The reality is that poor health, disease and illness progress slowly. We actually accumulate our sickness with dysfunctions in combinations of stress to our physical mental and chemical status. An inability of the body to cope with any or all of our balance leads to disease. The nervous system is responsible for managing all the other systems in the body and helping it cope or balance the stress. The central nervous system is responsible for managing all the other systems in the body and helping it cope or balance the stress. The central nervous system is housed in the brain and spinal cord, which are protected, by the skull and spine. When stresses are overwhelming the nervous system can be over taxed it. This condition is designated as a vertebral subluxation. Chiropractors devote their lives to correcting these subluxations with specific gentle adjustments to the spine column. There are times that a single adjustment may restore a great deal of balance back to the body but it is rate that one treatment will compensate for a lifetime of stress to an individual. It is more common that the number of treatments or necessity for care is in direct proportion to the length of time the body has been ill or the intensity of the exposure to stress. We suffer with the accumulation of micro-traumas coupled with macro traumas. An example would be a secretary seated all day in an awkward position (micro stress) who gets into car accident on her way home (macro stress).

Long-standing subluxations cause scar tissue or fibrosis to build up around the spinal discs, nerves and joints. These long-standing subluxations cause postural changes and tender muscle areas called trigger points. You may feel fine until someone touches these "hot" spots. This scar tissue takes a long time to heal and it may take months or years of spinal adjustments before your spine is strong again. The earlier you begin Chiropractic care the better: the longer you wait the greater the scar tissue accumulation and longer it will take to resolve.

Quote of the week: *"The earth is about five thousand million years old. Who can afford to live in the past?"*—Harold Pinter

Knee joint is complicated

Question: My knee pain has been getting progressively worse for one year. Now my hip, low back and ankle are hurting. Can the knee joint be the cause of this?

Answer: The knee is a very complicated joint. Its structure is supported by anterior and posterior collateral ligaments as well as medial and lateral collateral ligaments. The joint itself has a thin fluid lined surface called a meniscus. This allows for the smooth gliding action to the joint. Besides the meniscus and ligaments there are overlying tendons from muscles above and below on both the front and back of the leg. Above the joint the hamstrings attach in the posterior and the quadriceps attach in the anterior. Below the joint are the gastrocnemius attachments on the posterior and the anertior tibialis in the front. There is even an additional muscle behind the knee called the popliteal, which plays an important role in knee function. The reason I am giving you an anatomy lesson is to let you see how difficult it can be to find the specific cause of knee pain.

Even with the high potential to derange any one of these supportive tissues surrounding the knee, I find that the knee is more commonly a secondary adaptation to stresses elsewhere in the body. Chiropractors are very concerned with the biomechanics of the entire body and observe entire body posture and movements to determine the true cause of conditions. I find that although the patient may often complain of knee pain, a good portion of the time it is from an imbalance in their spine or pelvis. Adjusting the knee along with all other biomechanical imbalances will many times take stress off the soft tissue structures described in our anatomy lesson. Soft tissue will heal. Occasionally medication or surgery is required in severe tears and trauma. I suggest a complete and thorough evaluation by a Chiropractor that works with sports injuries and or extremities as a primary choice to determine the cause of your condition.

Quote of the week: *"The answers aren't important really…what's important is—knowing all the questions."*—Zilpha Keatley Snyder

Magnets may help back pain

Question: Do magnets help with chronic low-back pain? I have heard opposite opinions on this subject and understand there are all different kinds of companies and magnets. Do they work?

Answer: The use of magnets for back pain alone is more than a $5 billion industry in worldwide sales, with low-back pain the number one area of involvement marketed. Low-back pain is a disabling, costly condition. It is estimated that 85 percent of all people will have low-back pain during their lifetime. Currently, more than five million Americans are disabled with low-back pain.

The direct cost of treating low-back pain is estimated at $15 billion dollars annually. Bipolar magnets supposedly draw blood to the surface by attracting iron in the blood. The increase in vascular concentration draws minerals and vitamins found in the blood to the injured area. By engorging the damaged area with healing elements over a period of time, the process acts as a therapeutic treatment. Most recommended treatment with the magnets on the low back suggest six hours a day for at least three days a week.

Dr. Edward A. Collacott of the Veterans Affairs Medical Center, Prescott, Arizona, and his colleagues compared the effectiveness of one type of therapeutic bipolar magnet with a corresponding placebo device in 20 patients with chronic low-back pain. The results did not show a significant difference between the two. Other studies performed by magnet manufacturers indicate much more successful results.

My observation of patients who use magnet therapy indicates a definite relief of their chronic pain, but I don't believe it corrects the condition. I do know that if you want the cause of your low-back pain to be determined, you should first seek the advice of a Chiropractor. Chiropractors are trained to determine the causes of spinal conditions and correct them.

Quote of the week: *"It takes courage to grow up and become who you really are."*—e.e. cummings

Men and women must lift weight properly

Question: Are women more susceptible to low back pain from lifting heavy weight than men?

Answer: Women are obviously created physically different than men. Men are muscular and bone structures are thicker and denser in most cases. I know most of you women would agree, so are their brains. This may explain it.

A study printed in *Spine* magazine on November 15, 2002 explored the effects of spine loading as a function of gender. Two separate experiments on lifting performance were evaluated on 140 subjects. Electromyography assisted testing was utilized to determine spine loading during lifting performance.

The conclusion of the study indicated that woman are at a greater risk of muscoskeletal overload during lifting tasks. Individual body masses and pre-existing structural and functional postures play a role in how weight is distributed onto weight bearing structures of the body.

Proper preparation and intelligence prior to lifting is very prudent for either gender. Simple rules apply. Keep the weight close to your body. Keep your spine straight and lift with your legs. Intelligence will always succeed over brawn even in normal functional daily living tasks.

Quote of the week: *"Duty is a matter of the mind. Commitment is a matter of the heart."*—Anonymous

Mental exercises minimize senile dementia

Question: What can I do to stop loosing my mind? I am only 60 and I think I have senile dementia or Alzheimer's disease. I can't remember things told to me minutes prior and I have lapses of forgetting what I was going to do in the middle of a task?

Answer: Every person over the age of 60 should begin to think about his/ her cognitive function. This means staying alert with quick response and maintaining a good memory. Mental sharpness can slip away and someday; you're as bright as a vegetable. It doesn't have to be like this. Aging with an active mind can be far more creative than young minds because you have time to focus without all the diversions that young people have.

I have observed, even in the young teenagers, the exact same symptoms you describe in your question. In fact, I personally become brain dead on a regular basis according to my children. What I see and they observe are truly overloads of information and tasks upon the brain at one time. Our minds are overwhelmed with incomplete tasks and short circuit. The average parent has multi-task jobs on a daily basis. They are a taxi service for transportation, remembering schedules, a chef that cooks healthy meals and must shop for all the ingredients, a psychologist that must listen to all their families concerns, not to mention run a household and keep a job with a multitude of responsibilities including finances, health care, deadlines etc. It isn't a wonder that occasional early senility will occur. The best approach to recovering your wits is to breathe, relax and smell the flowers. The mind is an organ just like your heart or kidneys. It needs a rest once in a while. Meditation, Yoga and mental relaxation through relaxing activity such as reading a book can decompress the overload.

In your case, at 60 years old, where you may not have the sensory over-load and crazy emotional demands the opposite holds true. Many seniors stop a majority of their activities and let their minds stagnate. They don't allow for creative stimulation and get into very regular monotonous habits. To avoid this dysfunction that may lead to senile dementia it is imperative to exercise your mind. Join a club or organization to interact with other people. Try new hobbies or take classes in an area you never knew any-thing about. The brain cells are yearning for growth and inspiration.

Senile dementia can be the result of disease or genetic coding. There are multitudes of nutritional elements that claim they can prevent the onset of these symptoms. Some help some people and some do nothing for them. It is very individual. In severe cases a trained physician should be con-sulted.

Quote of the week: *"If you don't have wrinkles, you haven't laughed enough."*—Phyllis Dillar

Minds can create disease

Question: Is there such a thing as self-induced disease? My husband says he has SARS and he hasn't left the area in over a year.

Answer: Psychosomatically induced disease is very real. My original experience with this was as a student. Different classmates would contract the exact disease we were studying. While visualizing all the symptoms and physical effects of a syndrome, our brains can physically display the changes inside the body or as it is pictured in the brain. If an individual believes they have a condition they will get the condition.

I also had a very close relative whose sister and mother died at the age of 42 from uterine cancer. She went to her gynecologist every year for a check up to make sure she was healthy. She obsessed over the fear of getting this cancer. There was never a time I spoke with her that it wasn't mentioned. At 41 years of age, after being totally healthy for eight years of prior check ups, she was diagnosed with uterine cancer. She died of uterine cancer at age 42. Was this self induced or genetically predestined? We will never know.

I believe a healthy person requires positive mental focus, and a firm belief in their own body. The body was designed to be well and combat disease. Reorganizing our command center (brain and nervous system) to activate disease by envisioning the destructive behaviors of our environment can and will destroy normal healthy function in the body.

My advice is to have your husband focus on the positive aspects of the media and his environment. He requires a distraction from his obsession on the illness. If he has continued real symptoms he should seek a specialist in the healing field to assist him with his problem.

Quote of the week: *"Take each day and relish each moment. Take each bad day and work to make it good."*—Lisa Dade

Minor aches and pains can add up

Question: I have had a minor neck ache for over a year. It sometimes goes away on its own. Recently, all I did was fall asleep on the couch and woke up with my neck in severe pain. Could my recent odd sleeping position cause such a bad problem, or is this something that developed over time?

Answer: Your neck problem could be caused by many potential sources. You are correct in assuming the prior history of minor neck pain could lead to severe problems when unattended to properly. Most patients only consider their most recent experience of pain and the present time experience in their life. Many patients blame their pain on simple daily functions such as cleaning their homes, bending to brush their teeth or even sleeping oddly on their couch. These are usually the final episodes of a series of developing micro-traumas and stresses finally expressing themselves.

Our daily lives are full of various physical, mental, chemical, familial and sociological stresses. It is common for people to bare the ill effects of these stressors in their neck and trapezins region. By the end of the day, I see many patients and random people with their shoulders up to their ears.

Your neck has a tough enough job as it is. The cervical spine, made of seven small vertebra, has the job of holding up and balancing a 10-pund head. The movements of these vertebral joints are dependent on the function of dozens of intricately intertwined but perfectly placed muscles and ligaments.

Damaging your neck occurs when you fatigue or traumatize the muscles, ligaments or cervical joints. General causes of neck pain include sustained awkward positions, sleeping upright in a chair, overwork, slumping over a desk (especially a computer), carrying heavy suitcases or objects, or scrunching a telephone receiver between your ear and shoulder. Mental stresses such as anger, depression or fear tighten neck muscles leading to spasms and pain.

It is true that the recuperative healing powers of the body will correct mild neck sprains and strains. Persistent mild spasms, strains and pains, or severe trauma to your neck should be evaluated by a professional. Chiropractors are capable of examining and X-raying your cervical spine to determine the cause and degree of damage. Chiropractors use gentle treatment to reduce pain, improve range of motion, and restore normal function. Daily exercise and using proper body mechanics in your daily home and work routines will minimize your potential neck pain in the future.

Quote of the week: *"In dreams and in love there are no impossibilities."*—Janos Aranay

More study needed to manage kids' pain

Question: My child has constant pain in his joints. He suffered a severe trauma in a bicycle accident two years ago and he still has pain. Why would a child continue to have pain for so long?

Answer: In previous years a child's chronic pain was an enigma and never understood. Children are usually very resilient and recuperative when healing from trauma or injury. Physicians often times had expectations of nature correcting these chronic pain conditions because many do heal themselves with time. Recent research suggests that pain response in children has many potential factors. New research findings from laboratory and clinical studies have clearly identified possible mechanisms and provided evidence that long-term behavioral changes can extend far beyond what would be considered the normal long-term post-injury recovery. Timing, degree of injury, and administered analgesia and its nature may be important determinants of the long-term outcome of infant and child pain. The assessment and treatment of this pain and its functional consequences present a considerable unmet challenge.

In our Chiropractic clinic, we treat many of these chronic pain conditions in children. Our results have been outstanding in relationship to patient satisfaction regarding their pain reduction.

I will often listen to parents describe their child's pain as "growing pains." When the pains last months to years, it is hard to conceive of the condition being a growing pain. There truly is no condition called "growing pains."

Pain is a symptom or a protective mechanism of the body alerting you that you should attend to it immediately. Pain is usually the last sign you receive before more serous responses occur.

I suggest you do not ignore pain and have your child checked by a chiropractor or take him to a pediatrician who has a background in pain management and who will take a conservative approach to helping him.

Quote of the week: *"You never find yourself until you face the truth. "*—Pearl Bailey

Multidiscipline treatment for low-back pain coming of age

Question: I noticed your office and many other Chiropractic offices are offering multidiscipline treatment for back and other conditions. Could you explain what this type of approach to health care is?

Answer: I used to get the question why don't Chiropractors, medical doctors, and physical therapists get along, on a weekly basis. It is wonderful that society is recognizing the shift of new age healthcare. I do believe all health disciplines offer an integral part of the healthcare picture for you the patient. Combining these different approaches and utilizing the best expertise of each discipline offers the consumer a well-rounded viewpoint on the most successful treatment of their condition. The tricky part is organizing the disciplines in a most effective and cost efficient manner.

A recent study actually took a look at "Multidisciplinary Treatment of Chronic Low Back Pain". The results published in *Spine* magazine, April 2004 issue, concluded that long-term outcomes were very favorable for those studied. Past studies indicated definite improvement for short-term treatments of low back pain with the multi-disciplinarian approach.

There are many different combinations of the multi-discipline approach. Most include a more conservative type discipline such as Chiropractic, massage therapy, exercise physiologist, along with a more moderate type discipline such as physical therapy, acupuncture, or medical care. A successful model includes all those involved working as a team for your benefit.

Communication between the disciplines is imperative for understanding the needs of the patient. Many of these clinics are set up differently regarding insurance billing and financial responsibility. All these considerations should be explained to you in detail prior to treatment.

Progress is being made rapidly for the benefit of the patient. It would be nice if the insurance industry would recognize the benefits and cost containment these multidiscipline centers offer.

Quote of the week: *"Life consists in what a man is thinking all day."*—Ralph Waldo Emerson

Multiple diagnostic procedures
assist accuracy

Question: What is a MRI and CAT Scan and why would I get one done instead of X-rays?

Answer: Diagnostic-testing utilizing modern technology is expanding at a fast pace. The original static X-ray discovered by German physicist Dr. Wilhelm Roetgen in 1895, revolutionized the health-care field by allowing practitioners to identify pathology in bone tissues. As the "X-ray" evolved it became clearer and well defined in its assistance to health-care providers. The soft tissues such as ligaments and muscles could be differentiated in some cases and along with cross diagnostics in examination, became very helpful in differentially diagnosing conditions.

Radiographic images (X-ray) take a single moment in time and expose that structure onto a permanent imprint. The original X-ray was only productive for a one-dimensional view at a time. Most X-rays require a series of films taken to be considered a successful study.

X-rays next evolutionary step involved multiple single picture X-rays in series. This is called video fluoroscopy. Motion of a joint or bone can be observed using this method. The downfall of X-ray is the exposure to radiographic isotopes, which can be harmful to the body when excess exposure occurs. Video flutoscopy involves large doses of exposure.

The next invention to utilize picture of the internal body was computerized tomography (CT or CAT) scan. CTs allow the health-care practitioner to view various slices and angles with multi-dimensional views of the tissues in concern. Many times what was missed on an X-ray could be observed on CT scan. Once again, this diagnostic tool had the health consideration of radiation exposure.

The most modern technology, magnetic radiographic imaging (MRI) has no radiation exposure. The images are very clear and also allow multiple dimensions of the bone tissue and surfaces to be observed. No one diagnostic tool serves as a pure means for finalizing the cause of a condition. Careful physical examination, associated testing, bone scans, and other testing are the most accurate means of differentially diagnosing a condition.

In Chiropractic practices we primarily utilize static X-ray views. When any condition, especially a musculo-skeletal one, has any potential for severe disease that is outside of our practice it is proper protocol to refer out for an MRI, CT, bone scan or a combination of these diagnostic tests. A common condition we see in Chiropractic offices that requires the assistance of a MRI or CT of the spine are the conditions of a herniated or bulging vertebral disc. Static X-rays give us a good idea if these conditions exist, but MRI and CT are much more accurate to differential diagnose them. Once again, the best results occur from multiple diagnostic procedures.

Quote of the week: *"How things look on the outside of us depends on how things are on the inside of us. Remember, there is nothing wrong with nature, the trouble is in ourselves."*—Parks Cousins

Needlepoint and crocheting require posture consciousness

Question: For Christmas I do a lot of needlepoint preparing gifts for my family. When I finish my neck and shoulders are very sore. What do you suggest for stopping my pain?

Answer: You can control a lot of your potential discomfort yourself. Review your work area prior to doing your tasks. If it is possible, bring your materials closer to your head so you don't have to bend your neck as far forward. Also keep your materials within arms length distance away from your body so you don't have to reach as far causing over stretching of your arms and shoulders. I am sure you get very absorbed in your creations and may find yourself working at it for hours. Remind yourself to take breaks approximately every half an hour. Walk around, stretch your neck and shoulders by doing gentle neck ranges-of-motion and shoulder rolls forward and backward. Many needlepoint and crochet type designers also get wrist, hand and finger irritations from the fine movements that are demanded for these activities. Gentle stretching of the fingers and wrists periodically can reduce strain and sprain.

Should you continue to get persistent irritation in your neck, shoulders, arms, wrists or hands I suggest you consult a Chiropractor to determine if there is a condition that warrants treatment. Chiropractors are trained in analyzing, diagnosing and gentle treating most initial irritations in these areas. Don't wait for your symptoms to get worse. By the time you get your symptom you are already in trouble. The symptom is the last sign to show up and first to go away. Masking your pains with medications may hide the true cause of your problem and create a much worse condition in the future.

Quote of the week: *"The winds of grace are blowing all the time. You have only to raise your sail."*—Ramakrisna

New statistics are more accurate for children's normal growth indexes

Question: I am confused as to whether my 2-year-old is growing properly. His weight is lighter than most children his age and the information available shows dramatic differences in normal ranges. What is normal body weight for my son and should I be concerned?

Answer: If your son is healthy and asymptomatic most likely he is fine. A child's normal body weight can be affected by many factors including; genetic disposition, family eating habits, illness history, birth conditions and many other variables.

Previously, old but still widely used growth charts to determine "normal" weight and height for children were developed in the 1970s, on mostly white middle-class, formulated infants.

Presently, new charts have been developed by nutritionists, pediatricians and statisticians from the National Center for Health Statistics, the National Institute of Health and the Centers for Disease Control and Prevention where the old charts were based on just over 10,000 kids in Ohio. The new charts were based on national data on millions of diverse children. The new charts also take into account a child's body mass index rather than just weight. The old, or inaccurate charts, led to problems when expensive clinical tests were ordered for a healthy child that fell outside the growth chart. More information and the new growth charts can be found at www.cdc.gov/growthcharts.

Quote of the week: *"Act as though it were impossible to fail."*—Anonymous

Nutritional advice compliments Chiropractic care

Question: Why might my Chiropractor make dietary or nutritional recommendations as part of my treatment for back pain?

Answer: Keeping a healthy diet is always part of a holistic approach to health care for any patient. When a patient presents himself or herself with a severe acute condition or even a long-term chronic one, it is immediately understood that their body is being overtaxed for additional healing minerals and vitamins. Recovery from acute spinal injuries and chronic strain requires proper treatment from your Chiropractor and that treatment includes the building blocks to enhance healing in the form of proteins, vitamins, and minerals. For example, ligaments, muscles, and other tissues affected by spinal injuries and strains need additional vitamins such as B and C, as well as minerals like zinc, manganese, magnesium, and calcium to heal optimally. Your Chiropractor will also recognize the need for any additional nutrients that may be necessary depending on your unique physical dietary circumstances. Helping to build stronger, healthier muscle, ligaments, discs, bones and nerves to help your current condition improve and to gain better health through your lifetime is naturally an important duty of your Doctor of Chiropractic.

Quote of the week: *"Do the common thing in an uncommon way."*—Booker T. Washington

Observation best for determining child's health

Question: What should I look for and how will I know when to take my child to a Chiropractor?

Answer: Observation is the best method of determining if there may be a health problem with your child. Very young infants or newborns cannot express discomfort or point to an area that hurts. It is also difficult to distinguish cries of true basic needs as compared to a cry of pain. A child two or older can communicate their needs both verbally and non-verbally. It may not always be a parent that observes changes in a child. A teacher, childcare provider, or another trusted adult may be able to confirm potential abnormal changes.

Pain is not the only signal of a problem; in fact it is usually the last sign of a long developing condition. Leaving a problem unreported or unnoticed can be more difficult to be corrected by a Chiropractor than having your child checked regularly to avoid problems.

It is a great habit for any parent or childcare giver to observe children: running, jumping, walking, sitting, standing and at play. These moments when the child is most unselfconscious, unaware that anyone is watching, will yield the most accurate information. Observe your child's posture for asymmetries in their body, skull, extremities, skull and spine. Observe these same structures when your child is active.

Your child's emotional state may reveal information about a problem that the child may not be aware of. Look for irritability, unusual emotional sensitivity, or changes in eating habits, sleeping patterns, and play patterns.

If your observations of your child's posture, emotional state, or behaviors indicate a problem call your Doctor of Chiropractic to discuss your concerns. Your Chiropractor will help you determine if there is a chance your child could benefit from a Chiropractic examination and treatment. The only person that can determine that your child has a condition that would benefit from Chiropractic care is your Doctor of Chiropractic. When in doubt, simply call.

Quote of the week: *"Children are likely to live up to what you believe of them."*—Lady Bird Johnson

Organic produce is more nutritious

Question: I have heard a lot of hype about produce having little nutritious value. Is it true that organic produce is more nutritious than standard fruits and vegetables?

Answer: You have probably noticed that almost every grocery store in Ocean County has an organic food or natural food section if not both. You now have a choice as to which produce to consume. Organic produce is more beneficial nutritionally than standard produce. Organic produce usually tastes better, has not been genetic all altered, and is less likely to contain chemical fertilizers. The bottom line is that organic produce contains more nutrients.

A study in the British Food Journal compared the 1930s' nutrient content of 20 fruits and vegetables with foods grown in the 1980s. Significant reductions were found in the levels of calcium, copper, and magnesium in vegetables, and magnesium, iron, copper and potassium in fruit. Similar trends can be found in foods produced in the United States, with reductions in some nutrients as much as 32 percent.

A recent study by Dr. Virginia Worthington, while at John Hopkins University, showed that vitamins C, iron, magnesium and phosphorus were higher inorganic grown foods.

There are numerous certifies organic farms in our area that sell healthier organic produce at a reasonable price, comparable to standard produce in large super market chains.

The best way to get organic produce is to grow it yourself. With just a little yard space you can grow a small vegetable plot. Properly tended you can yield enough vegetables in season to feed your entire family. By growing your own vegetable you can ensure the quality, reduce costs and reel in the enjoyment of producing your own food, not to mention the extra exercise you get working in your garden.

Quote of the week: *"He who laughs at himself, always has the last laugh."—Anonymous*

Parents have the magic touch

Question: I recently gave birth to a 7-week premature baby and want to know if what I observed is common. When my baby was held and touched by me, my husband or even the nurses, I could see and feel positive changes in my baby. His temperature improved; his color flushed and his breathing normalized. Is it possible that just human touch can heal?

Answer: There is tremendous power in the human touch for all living beings. Babies thrive on touch and adults are not too far behind.

A new study published in *Pediatrics* states that babies with low birth weight benefit from skin-to-skin contact. When compared to infants in incubators, newborns with skin-to-skin contact had less severe infections, spent fewer days in the hospital and had better head circumferences, a sign of better growth rate.

The system discussed above involves placing a diaper-clad preemie upright on his mom's bare chest, tummy to tummy, in between her breasts, inside her clothing; her body warmth helps stabilize the baby's temperature and also allows for easier breast-feeding.

The system is now being implemented in neonatal clinics in the United States, Canada, and Europe. The moms also claim a sense of empowerment with the touch of their baby against their skin.

Another story I recently read discussed the grim chances of a palm-sized twin born in a remote village hospital. All her vital signs were unstable and her chances of survival were grim. Due to a shortage of beds, the baby was placed with her infant twin in the same bed. Immediately the twins snuggled up close together. The unstable sibling made significant improvement and slept for the first time. In the hours and days that ensued, the frail baby stabilized, survived and became healthy. During that period the siblings stayed close at all times.

Babies and adults are proof of the wondrous healing power of the strongest of all medicines—touch.

Quote of the week: *"When you're drawing up your first list of miracles, you might place near the top the first moment your baby smiles at you."*—Bob Green

Patients can help in the healing process

Question: How can I assist my Chiropractor in helping with the correction of my spinal problems?

Answer: There are many ways in which you can assist your Chiropractor with the healing process and maintenance of your spine and nervous system.

1. Have confidence in your Chiropractor's decisions and treatment. Being aligned with the same goals and strategies for your best potential health provides a sense of team effort.

2. Drink plenty of water. Consuming six large eight-ounce glasses of water daily provides enough water to nurture your muscles and organ systems as well as flush out toxins.

3. Stretch daily. Allow motion to joints to move fresh blood supply through all your tissues enhancing the bodies natural healing processes. Yoga is a wonderful mind-body balancing stretching art that supports spinal functions.

4. Minimize exposure to toxins into your body. Eat intelligently, avoiding excess sugars, empty carbohydrates, fried-fatty foods, artificial colorings, pesticides, and chemicals. Avoid smoking or smoky environments. Reduce alcohol and or drugs if they are habits.

5. Communicate openly with your Chiropractor. Let him or her know of any stressful changes in your life or any positive results of the treatment.

6. Keep a positive outlook on life. Read or watch inspirational and motivational books and movies. Avoid the negativity of TV newscasts and commercialized advertising.

7. Meditate or rest your mind daily so it doesn't get overtaxed.

8. Laugh out loud and laugh a lot. Life is short so find the things in life that are fun and indulge.

9. Be responsible for your life and health and don't blame any misfortune on others or become a victim.

Quote of the week: *"Success doesn't come to you…you go to it."*—Marva Collins

Plane travel can be comfortable

Question: I am an airplane passenger three or more days a week. I get extremely sore backaches after my flights. Could you suggest ways I could reduce or eliminate my pain?

Answer: Flying first class, while receiving a massage with warm moist towels on your face would make your flights much less stressful. Unfortunately, the reality is that we must fit our butts into tiny seats with our knees squished up to our abdomen. While imprisoned in your undersized child seat you must keep your body still with your seatbelt securing you in place. Keep your elbows close to your body to make sure you don't poke your fellow sardine next to you. Now try to read a book, write a novel, or conduct business on your laptop. I must admit, you have an uphill battle to defeat the air flight experience.

I am supposed to give you advice and solutions so here is what I suggest. Take the bus. Only kidding. Preparation prior to flying is very helpful. Stretch your entire body. Yoga is extremely fruitful for compensating the joints of the body and relaxing your mind. Cardiovascular exercise 2 to 3 times weekly will keep your heart and lungs healthy, compensating for the stagnant positions you are forced to maintain.

Carry a neck support pillow on flights to support your head. Avoid falling asleep with your head flopping off to one side. Get out of your seat as often as possible, only when the "safe to move around the cabin" light is on of course. Simple neck ranges of motion, shoulder shrugs along with shoulder forward and backward rolls can be done seated or standing.

Drink plenty of water. Flight travel dehydrates the body and is a major cause of joint pain. Avoid heavy carry on bags that stress the neck and shoulders. In the meantime sit up straight and enjoy your flights.

Quote of the week: *"A certain amount of opposition is a great help to a person. Kites rise against, not with the wind."*—John Neal

Positive happy staff help keep Chiropractic offices busy

Question: I recently moved back to New Jersey and have now been to four different Chiropractors around the country. All their offices seem upbeat and positive compared to medical offices I have visited. What makes Chiropractic offices so happy compared to other healing facilities?

Answer: Different healing arts attract different patients. Many medical healing arts contend with death, dying and illness. Chiropractic on the contrary deals with life, living and wellness. It is definitely easier to be upbeat in the second scenario. There must be chemistry between the patients; the doctor's staff, the doctors and the environment that the healing is taking place in. An upbeat staff that smiles and shows genuine concern for their patients makes a great first impression. Communication between all parties involved in a healing facility is essential for success.

In any business, quality service with a smile adds to the level of satisfaction of the consumer. In the health industry it is more than just a service, it is essential to the healing process. I believe that Chiropractors and their natural healing philosophy manifest itself in the way they treat their staff, family and patients. Most Chiropractors I have encountered, myself included, practice what they preach. When a physician of any type has a passion for what they do and truly believe in their work it is self-evident. There are many levels of healing that occur when two people interact, especially a doctor and their patient. There is the intellectual level, the physical level and the spiritual level. If any portion of the connection is not accepted or conflicted a gap may occur that does not allow healing to occur.

To answer your question, Chiropractors offices seem happier and more upbeat because most of them comprehend the value of satisfying their patients needs on all planes. A content patient that feels their problems were attended to, and not even necessarily corrected, will still be happier and more fulfilled. The feeling that someone or an entire office sincerely cares is contagious and people tend to want to share that with their friends and family. This is why many Chiropractic officers are busy. Happy offices are self-perpetuating.

Quote of the week: *"Some people dream of worthy accomplishments, while others stay awake and do them."*—Anonymous

Posture evaluation is best for determining spinal dysfunction

Question: When I look in the mirror at myself I notice my shoulder is much higher on the left than the right and my one hip is higher on the opposite side. I get constant neck, shoulder and low-back pain. What do these changes in my posture indicate and are they related to my symptoms?

Answer: Posture is the most pure identification of adaptive changes to stress in the body. Ideally, your posture should be symmetrical from your head to your toes. Your head should be centered directly over your shoulders with no forward or backward tilt. Check one ear in relationship to the other to determine head tilt. Your shoulders should be on an even plane without forward rotation or rounded posture. Your navel should be centered in the middle of your torso in relationship to your midline from your chin to the ground. Hips should be even height without one rotating forward or backward. Your knees should be facing forward and balanced from one to the other. Excessive internal or external rotation is not a normal posture. Your feet and ankles should be forward and even just as the knees are. The feet are an excellent determinant of poor weight bearing in the body and indicate just where the inappropriate forces are being redirected. When an evaluation is made of all the components of postural distortion a clear and precise diagnosis of the cause of a structural condition can be made. Combine the postural evaluation with a good history of the patient and the majority of the approach to correct the condition should be evident. Since structure and function are inseparable, correcting the structural condition can directly help the functional disorder.

An important factor to remember when looking at posture is that no matter how your body distorts itself the eyes will always be straight and the feet will touch the ground. This may seem self evident, but if you under-stand this then you will realize that all the other distortions in your posture are righting mechanisms to compensate for gravity pressing down on us all day. Unfortunately the greatest brunt of weight-bearing imbalance is gen-erated to the spine where sensitive nerve tissue immediately responds send-ing impulses to muscles to balance us. A repetitive or individually severe response to the muscles results in spasms. This response is why you may get pain in various related joints such as your neck, low back, shoulders, etc.

I suggest you evaluate yourself in the mirror and objectively review your own posture. A Chiropractor is trained to know exactly what each distor-tion indicates and can treat you as well as educate you on how some or all of these changes may be corrected.

Quote of the week: *"The journey of a thousand miles starts with a single step."*—Chinese proverb

Power of threes helps self-discipline

Question: I am a single mom raising two young boys, ages 11 and 13, and find it difficult to communicate to them the importance of posture and health. I know you treat children. Could you suggest any methods to help me to help them?

Answer: When I stated out I practice 23 years ago someone gave me a small short book called the "Power of Threes." The book claimed that if you desire something (anything) you could make it come true by focusing on it constantly. The book implied that discipline, clarity of desire and repetition could allow your dreams and goals to come true. I must tell you it works. It worked for me 23 years ago and still does today. These are the action steps to create a solution to the frustration in communicating with your children regarding personal health care.

First, get very clear on exactly what you want your outcome to be. Write out all the sensory attachments and precise results and how it will make you feel when accomplished. Reduce it all to one or two sentences. For example: "I will communicate successfully to my children by daily conversation and demonstrations on how to be healthier. We will all be happier and healthier."

Write it down and post it in places you will see throughout the day—the mirror in your bathroom, your car, your refrigerator or desk at work. Here is where the "Power of Threes" starts. Read your goal three times, say it out loud three times and tell three people, minimum, daily what your goal is. It is OK to do it more than three times. After a while your mind and body will attract a solution to your goal and it will come true.

A large part of gaining respect and achievement from children is respecting yourself and demonstrating your own commitment and integrity. Children may initially give resistance but will usually follow a good role model such as a parent.

Quote of the week: *"When integrity meets creativity, vision naturally grows."*—Pat McHenry Sullivan

Preparation prevents neck pain at the computer

Question: My job requires me to spend hours a day in front of a computer. My neck pain has gotten worse to the point it hurts all day and night. I can't give up my job, so what can I do?

Answer: Improper computer positioning can definitely contribute to neck pain. The best solution to preventing further irritation is to give your work site an ergonomic study. Step back from your work site and examine the location of all your equipment. Here is a checklist of items to review:

1. Make sure that your chair, desk, table and workstation are at the right height for you. If more than one person will be using the same equipment, make it easy to adjust to each person.

2. Position your computer so it is at eye level or just below eye level. You do not want to be looking up at the screen, and you do not want to be looking down at a sharp angle.

3. Keep all your paperwork as close to eye level as possible. There are many stands available that allow paperwork to be placed next to computer monitors and prevent having to turn your head back and forth from paperwork to monitor.

4. Take frequent breaks. Get up, stretch tired muscles, and allow your eyes to focus on something in the distance. Doing this will help prevent eye and neck strain as well as headache.

5. Use a telephone headset if you spend long hours on the phone while also at the computer. Cradling the phone between your ear and shoulder quickly tires muscles and creates tension.

6. Breathing and relaxation exercises throughout the day help keep your focus and reduce mental and physical stress.

7. Examine other areas of your life that may stress your neck. Common problem areas include poor postures while sleeping, reading, or watching television in bed, driving in your car, lifting objects or children and many more.

Most importantly to avoid recurrent episodes of neck pain follow all of your Doctor of Chiropractic's instructions for healing and prevention. Chiropractors can examine and diagnose the cause of your neck pain. Using modern technology of X-rays and other specific testing your conditions cause can be determined so specific gentle corrections can be made. Healing is a dual effort and even though Chiropractic works it is your responsibility to make your own personal adjustments in your life activities to maintain your health and prevent injuries.

Quote of the week: *"Learning is discovering that something is possible."*—Fritz Perls

Preparation prevents water-sport injuries

Question: My family spends most of the summer doing water sports. It seems someone always gets an injury early in the season. How can we avoid water-sport injuries?

Answer: Swimming, water skiing, and boating are usually short outdoor seasons in New Jersey. We utilize muscles and move in positions we do not normally use throughout the prior seasons. When warm weather hits we have a tendency to over indulge without proper stretching and preparation. We see common early season injuries of shoulder strain, low-back and hip injuries, along with neck sprains/strains.

Water skiing injuries usually occur due to poor falling techniques. If you know you are going to fall let your entire body go limp. Let all your joints and muscles relax which minimizes the initial impact into the water. Boating accidents often occur getting into the boat as often as the bouncing and jostling from jumping the wakes. Avoid carrying coolers, towels, dogs, kids, and equipment all at once or while stepping into the boat. Make multiple trips and hand items to people inside the boat. As you are wave hopping across the water anticipate the waves and bumps. Hold onto stable parts of the boat, bend your knees, and move with the motion of the boat to absorb the shock from the watercraft into your spine.

Water sports should be safe and fun. Always take precautions with your equipment and check for proper function and safety. Always pre-plan your activities and know what and where to go in case of emergencies.

If injuries occur, take care of them as soon as possible and make sure to tell your Chiropractor of any falls or injuries whether you are experiencing symptoms or not. Appropriate and immediate care by a Chiropractor can expedite correction and healing.

Quote of the week: *"You can give without loving, but you cannot love without giving."*—Amy Carmichel

Psoas muscle keeps us standing

Question: I was told by my therapist that I had a psoas muscle problem. What does this muscle do and how is it related to my lower back pain?

Answer: Anatomicaly your psoas muscle inserts into the lower lumbar spine of the low back and attaches to the top and front of the hipbone on both sides of your pelvis. The two psoas muscles create a 45-degree angle as they descend from the lower spine and appear as two support structures holding the lower spine in place. Symmetry of these two muscles is imperative. When one muscle is more active or stronger than the other it will cause movement of the vertebra or hip to be out of alignment. The body will always attempt to right itself from a bent or crooked position. The spasm of these muscles can bend a person in various directions as a means of avoiding pain. This awkward positioning away from pain is called antalgia and is very common with psoas spasm syndromes.

The psoas muscles crucial role in maintaining our lumbar spine makes it susceptible to injury with many activities. The psoas main function as it contracts is to elevate the leg and turn the foot out especially in the initial phase of walking. A classic sign of psoas imbalance is pain that grabs in the anterior hip or low back as a person goes to stand up. Other symptoms include; pain, restriction or clicking in the acetabulum (hip joint), sciatica, female disorders, intestinal problems, kidney problems, poor circulation to the anterior thigh and legs, low back fatigue, achiness, and pain, knee and ankle problems as well as a limp.

Correction of the condition is a matter of reducing the psoas spasm on the hyperactive side and increasing the strength on the weaker side. Additionally, Chiropractic adjustments may be required to gently restore balance back to the vertebra and or hipbone. Deep massage and home exercise therapy are helpful in keeping the balance in these muscles.

Quote of the week: *"Anything in life is possible if you make it happen. And its never too late."*—Jack La Lanne

Referred pain is a serious protective signal

Question: I have been having pain under my right shoulder blade for weeks and I haven't done anything different in my daily activities and have not been in an accident. My back never hurt me in the past. Could my back pain be caused from a problem somewhere else in my body?

Answer: You are describing a potential mechanism in the body called referred pain. The body doesn't always elicit pain over the same area that a problem is occurring. Specific organs, muscles, glands, bones and soft tissues in the body carry common neurological and vascular supplies. The central nervous system controls and coordinates the activities of all the feedback loops from the interaction of all these different tissues. When there is a dysfunction of too much input or too little input in relationship to balanced activity the central nervous system will identify the source. One of the responses the CNS (central nervous system) may give is pain. It can be directly over the imbalanced tissue or it may be along the path of nerve or vascular distribution. The nerve and blood supply usually travel in tandem.

Understanding the anatomy, along with clinical studies of commonly referred areas of pain, helps physicians diagnose conditions. Your area of referred pain, under the right scapula, is associated with gall bladder or liver dysfunction. Additional differential diagnostic testing such as ultrasound and blood work, along with x-ray and physical examination could help isolate the true cause of your pain. Another classic initial indication in referred pain is severe mid-abdominal pain, which can imply a ruptured appendix. Metastasizing carcinomas will refer pain from their original source also. Many of these conditions are referred to the spine itself.

Chiropractors are trained to identify whether your back pain is structural versus organic and to know when there is an emergency potentially present. It is our job to refer you to the appropriate treatment source at this point. If your back pain is not referred or organic in nature then no one is better to treat you than your Chiropractor.

Quote of the week: *"Some men still have their first dollar. The man who is really rich is the one who still has his first friend."*—Anonymous

Remain true to resolutions

Question: In January I made all these great health resolutions and was really motivated. Now it is March and I am back to the same old patterns. What can I do to stay motivated?

Answer: You are not alone. Maintaining your motivation to stay healthy takes a strong conviction and focus. I have five suggestions to help you stick with it.

1. Don't make or agree to do a healthful habit that is totally against what you can do and like to do. This creates conflict within you. An example would be committing to jogging every day, when you hate jogging. You can get the same cardio-vascular workout with swimming and or biking.

2. Modify behaviors. Rather than create total chaos rearranging your daily routines to meet illusions of transformation, take gradual adjustments that build on each other. An example would be to change one meal a day to a healthy meal or remove one negative food from each meal daily until your entire diet is healthy.

3. Use positive reinforcement. Try the power of threes. Say what you want out loud three times daily, read it three times daily and tell three people daily. Use affirmative statements that support your healthy goals. An example would be to say, "I am losing five pounds because I feel terrific at that weight," as opposed to saying, "I am losing five pounds because I am fat."

4. Create a plan. The more organized and specific your plan is the more focused you will be. Review your progress each week and reward yourself.

5. Enlist support. Be open to help. Recruit a friend or family member as a support or join a group that shares your same objectives.

Quote of the week: *"You don't know how much you don't know until your children grow up and tell you how much you don't know."*—S.J. Perelman

Roller coaster rides could cause injuries

Question: My son wants me to go on the rides with him at the theme park. I am concerned about my spine. Is it safe to go on roller coaster type rides with a history of neck or back problems?

Answer: Many theme park rides are very traumatic to the body. We treat many patients that have had neck whiplash and low back sprain and strain injuries on rides.

This does not mean they are not safe. Most thrill rides require safety guidelines to prevent or minimize potential injuries to riders. Most rides have disclaimers on signs prior to riding, informing the public that they can create sudden and rapid movements to the body. Almost all rides inform potential riders that they should not get on if they are pregnant, suffer from heart conditions or have pre-existing medical conditions.

Your pre-existing condition of neck or low-back pain should be examined by a competent physician such as a Chiropractor to determine potential additional injury or exacerbation.

Spending time with your child doing something he or she enjoys, sometimes supercedes the fear of re-injuring your condition. Use common sense and if the ride looks like it is traumatic to the people on it, then avoid it. The most important idea is to have safe fun and quality time.

Quote of the week: *"Be grateful for luck but don't depend on it."*

Running extends life

Question: I have heard that running is both good and bad for your health. Is it healthy to run and what are its benefits?

Answer: A study in the journal *The Lancet* in November 2002 reviewed 370 members of a running club for people over 50. The study indicates that regular running may increase life expectancy and risk of disability in old age for an extended time of 9 years. Not only are deaths prevented, disability levels are decreased and the development of disability is postponed in association with running and other aerobic exercise.

Running of any moderate to intensity exercise performed four days or more a week for 45 minutes minimum may assist in the longevity and quality of life. A key to these positive results is combining your exercise with preventive measures. Always stretch before and after aerobic exercise, drink plenty of water and wear supportive well-made footwear.

Chiropractic is an imperative adjunct to a regular exercise program. Spinal balance minimizes potential injury and allows proper weight bearing distribution to the hips, knees, ankles, and feet. Running on an imbalanced pelvis or spine will overtax one or all of the above mentioned joints, leading to soft tissue or joint disturbance. Avoid running with injuries and have your spine checked prior to and during your aerobic workouts to maintain the highest potential of benefit from your exercise.

Quote of the week: *"The price of greatness is a responsibility."*—Anonymous

Scar tissue causes chronic pain

Question: Why do I still experience neck and shoulder pain years after my whiplash accident? I have had physical therapy and Chiropractic treatment without success. What would you suggest?

Answer: The main source of chronic joint irritation is fibrotic tissue development. Fibrotic tissue, also referred to as scar tissue, is much more dense and thick than healthy elastic tissue. Scar tissue develops within 24 hours of a trauma.

Our bodies attempt to heal damaged tissue from either an individual trauma or a series of micro-traumas by creating an inflammatory reaction. Inflammation is the body's natural healing process. It involves attracting fluid to injured tissue. The fluid contains minerals and vitamins and a matrix of healing elements designed to saturate the damaged area so it can absorb the nutrients and heal.

Inflamed tissue can resolve on its own but it will always leave behind a remnant of tissue thickening.

When we are younger the scar tissue doesn't seem to be a deterrent to movement or function. When we get into our mid-30s to mid-40s, the natural aging process adds additional thickening due to a slowing down of our elastic tissue production. Metabolism slows down, and so does repair time for injuries.

Former thickening coupled with normal aging can influence joint, muscle and ligament sensitivity due to restricted motion. The main tissue affected is the fascia (the paper-thin covering of a muscle). A wrinkled fascia over your muscle interferes with its normal contractions and leads to pain and dysfunction.

Chronic pain is predominately the result of thickened scar tissue and facial wrinkling. Many new protocols in massage therapy, physical therapy and Chiropractic care now focus on attending to this scar tissue phenomenon. The results have been astoundingly positive. We are successfully treating patients who did not respond in the past. Techniques vary among the different healing arts but all are beneficial.

Consider giving your condition some of the new technology and I believe your chronic pain could improve.

Quote of the week: *"Genius is the ability to reduce the complicated to the simple."*—C. W. Ceran

Shingles is difficult to diagnose

Question: I recently had severe pain in the middle of my back along my ribs that turned into a rash. It still hurts even two months later. I was told it was shingles. Why is it so painful and lasts so long?

Answer: Shingles is a herpes zoster virus similar to the virus identified in chicken pox. Your description of acute severe pain in the mid-back along the ribs is the most common nerve root region to be affected. Many patients will experience severe pain and some only slight pain. Most shingles conditions demonstrate a blistering rash that follows along the nerve's path, usually along the ribs in the back or chest. Another area that I have observed shingles in my patients is on the face. This is also a very sensitive and painful area. It is almost as common not to get a rash initially or at all, which makes it difficult to diagnose shingles. Many patients may have just a few red marks and no pain or minimal pain.

Why it is so painful and why it affects only certain people at certain times is still difficult to discern. My observation is that the patients that experience the herpes zoster virus are those that are under extreme stress or have just resolved a stressful condition. I believe a healthy lifestyle of eating wholesome foods, mental relaxation, physical exercise, and proper rest are helpful in minimizing the contraction of the virus. Maintaining a healthy immune system will definitely help predisposition to the virus as well as any virus.

Chiropractic has helped my patients with shingles by balancing the nervous system and directly effecting the immune system. I am always postulating why two people exposed to the same virus will react totally opposite, one contracting the virus while the other does not. Shingles falls into the same category as all the unknown causes of disease—the weakening of the immune system. Strengthen your nervous system with Chiropractic treatment and you will assist your immune system.

Quote of the week: *"If you've made up your mind you can do something, you're absolutely right."*—Anonymous

Singer voices Chiropractic results

Question: My music teacher goes to a Chiropractor to keep her voice in shape. How does a Chiropractor help your voice?

Answer: The nervous system has influence over every cell tissue and organ in the body including the throat.

Your voice requires multiple muscle groups to be functioning in order to produce various pitches, tones and volumes.

Singers can strain these muscles with over use exertion or improper breathing from the diaphragm. The sprained muscles of the throat are similar to any sprained muscles in your body. They swell, retain fluid and get sore. Initially, (first 48 hours) apply ice to reduce inflammation. Additional treatment involves muscle balancing as well as re-positioning of the hyoid bone, which is not directly attached to any other bones. Bones within the palate, specifically the sphenoid bone can effect voice functions. Also, commonly, the cervical spine will develop vertebral subluxations, which irritate nerve supply to the function of the throat and voice.

Chiropractors specialize in correction vertebral subluxations and that is why your music teacher seeks Chiropractic care to assist in correcting her voice condition.

Quote of the week: *"We may affirm absolutely that nothing great in the world has been accomplished without passion."*—George Wilhelm Friedrich Hesel

Sitting at work requires breaks

Question: I am stuck at work sitting at my computer for six or more hours a day. I feel sore all over by the end of my shift. What advice could you give me to reduce my pain, because I can't give up the job?

Answer: Millions of people who their living while sitting needlessly endure excessive pain, stress and strain, as they perform their daily tasks. These complaints are common among seated workers although they are not normal. Taking stress-reducing exercise breaks, along with thorough evaluation of your workspace and work environment, can make a tremendous positive improvement in your health.

Here are some tips that can commonly help the new high-tech seated computer worker.

- When using your keyboard, keep your elbows close to your body and your wrists parallel to the keyboard. This position reduces wrist strain and minimizes neck, shoulder and arm discomfort.

- Reduce eyestrain by changing your focus to an object in the distance or closing your eyes for 10 seconds. You can avoid headaches by checking the surrounding lighting and reflective glare from your monitor.

- Your head, neck and body should be squarely aligned with the height a position of your monitor so it is no tilted or rotated in any position for an extended time.

- Your chair should have a back support that is in contact with your low back. Your knees should be slightly higher than hips and your spine should be supported so it is held erect.

- Your feet should firmly touch the floor, or put a large book such as a phone book under one foot to keep the back firmly against the back of your chair.

- Taking a healthy stretch break is imperative to minimizing joint discomfort. Walk around, stretch and breathe deeply and slowly as you raise your hands over your head.

It is becoming a priority for companies across the country to implement programs to help workers become healthier and more productive. Take it upon yourself to make positive changes in your own work environment.

Quote of the week: *"In the end, what affects your life most deeply are the things too simple to talk about."*—Nell Blaine

Sleep position that is best for neck

Question: What is the best way to sleep with regard to the position of my neck and head? What is the best pillow to use?

Answer: The natural healthy curve in your neck is a "C" curve. Your neck's posture is designed to evenly distribute the weight bearing of your head against gravity pressing downward. When the neck is straight the weight is distributed to the lower cervical vertebra alone causing undue accumulative stress leading to arthritis and degeneration. When you lie flat on your back and your neck's curve is supported by a pillow without elevating the skull your "C" curve of your neck is stabilized and the muscles surrounding the spine are relaxed.

Lying on your side with your head turned to the side and the neck's curve supported is the second best position to sleep.

If you are a belly sleeper it is difficult to support the neck appropriately. My advice is to use no pillow at all in this scenario.

There are many specially designed cervical (neck) pillows that support the "C" curve in your neck. Some are firmer than others. It is the individuals' preference. There are also travel cervical pillows that support your neck while seated.

Ultimately, avoid pushing your head and chin forward toward your chest with a large pillow. Use a thin pillow or no pillow at all to allow the natural postural contours of your neck to be healthy.

Quote of the week: *"Make the most of today. Translate your good intentions into actual deeds."*—Grehulle Kleiser

Some Chiropractors make house calls

Question: I have had severe low-back pain and could not move out of my bed. I did not want to go to the emergency room. Had I called you or any Chiropractor would you have come to my house to treat me?

Answer: House calls do still exist. Yes, I do make them myself under absolute needy circumstances. Among my colleagues there is a mixed opinion as to performing house calls. Unfortunately, there is always a concern for liability reasons.

When the call is from an existing patient it is easier to differentially diagnose a need for care versus at-home therapy. I always try to avoid home visits because my experience is that the majority of the ones I performed were either unnecessary or truly an emergency situation that required an ambulance or hospital attention.

A new-patient house call is rare because I usually have no background or history prior to the treatment of the patient. Most times I can give advice over the phone until they can get mobile enough to get into my office. I have no problem with treating a new patient at a home visit as long as I can perform testing that can determine their status. Also, I avoid vicious pit bulls and untamed aggressive pets such as tigers and lions.

Our society has created rigid privacy controls that most people don't even request home visits anymore. Be assured that true caring and help is still available for the needy patient.

Quote of the week: *"The answer to having a better life is not about getting a better life, it's just about changing how we see the one we have right now."*—Angel Kyodo Williams

Stretching a must for weekend warrior

Question: I am a weekend warrior with sports. I play softball on the weekends and want to know if stretching really makes a difference?

Answer: The answer is a resounding yes, especially for the weekend warrior. You are typical of the average adult athlete. Whether it is two or seven days a week that you work out, stretching is imperative to prepare for activity, prevent injury and cool down muscles after working them.

It only takes approximately 15 minutes to appropriately stretch prior to physical activity. Stretching is essential because it elongates the muscles prior to use. An unprepared muscle that is given a rapid stretch will pull from its origin and insertion around the bone from which it attaches. The end points of muscles are tendons and their responsibility is to attach to bone. When the muscles vigorously pull at these tendons they move the bone to quickly causing a strain at this region. A strain is accompanied by swelling, restriction of movement and pain. Pre-stretching the muscle and tendons prepares the tissue for sudden, quick jolts by elongating the tendons' insertions. Pre-stretching prior to a jolt is less likely to cause a strain because there is more length to the tendon to adapt to the movement. Stretching also prevents injuries to the belly of the muscle. The belly of the muscle contains fluid. A cooler fluid moves slower and adapts slower to movement. Stretching warms out the stagnant cooler fluids in the belly and dissipates toxins such as lactic acid that accumulate secondary to dormancy.

A well-prepared muscle means a well-prepared joint. The joints that are predominantly used for your particular activity should be concentrated on, although full-body stretching is always recommended.

A well-prepared body includes a well-prepared nervous system. Many athletes choose Chiropractic care to enhance their performance. The nervous system controls muscle function and if you continue to feel tight or sore in your muscular regions you should consult a Chiropractor to determine if assistance is required.

Quote of the week: *"Failure is not the worst thing in the world…The very worst is not to try."*—Anonymous

Stroke unrelated to treatment

Question: I recently saw a news report on television that Chiropractic adjustments cause strokes. Is it true?

Answer: No, it is absolutely not true. The incidence of strokes caused by Chiropractic adjustments is less likely than getting hit by lightning. The archaic news stories you have seen are pure propaganda distributed by a disgruntled medical profession that is making a last gasp at survival by attacking Chiropractors.

I have written previous columns citing multiple studies, which accurately surveyed and studied the incidence of strokes caused directly by Chiropractors.

When analyzed it was determined that the strokes—the minute number of patients claimed to be caused by Chiropractors—were actually not from Chiropractors but from prior experiences or from other healing practitioners.

If Chiropractic were so dangerous, as the false claims suggest, you would think our malpractice rates would be sky high. On the contrary, Chiropractic is safe, gentle and effective. Our malpractice rates are 50 times less than the average medical physician's.

Patients would never consider bringing their babies and children to a Chiropractor if it were dangerous. The fact is parents do bring their kids in for primary health-care and personally it is rare that children get injured, let alone get strokes.

Shame on the medical profession for allowing such slander to be published and recorded. We already defeated their attacks in the 1980s by winning an anti-trust lawsuit. In the Wilkes vs. American Medical Association (AMA) case we—the Chiropractors—proved the AMA was attempting to defame the character of the Chiropractic profession by setting up an anti-quackery committee to distribute lies and defamation to destroy our profession.

Shame on the medical profession to isolate a rare unique occurrence in the Chiropractic field when iatrogenic (doctors-induced illness and death) is considered the third cause of death and illness in our country.

I suggest the medical public relations representatives put their wasted money back into the medical field to clean up their own mess before continually attacking other fellow healing professions.

Quote of the week: *"Get mad. Then get over it."*—Colin Powell

Structure is function and function is structure

Question: I find that when I am sick my body doesn't feel balanced and that after being bent over at work all day it makes me feel ill. Is there a relationship between my posture and my illness?

Answer: We have a saying in Chiropractic that goes like this: "Structure is function and function is structure." For every action by the body there is a direct reaction by the nervous system. For every change to the nervous system there is a direct effect to whatever body tissue that area of the nervous system enervates. An example of this would be a typical computer tech that is inputting data all day while seated. The technician's low back is receiving an over abundance of neurological input to right itself under all this continuous compressive force. In response to this pressure the nervous system must send constant signals to the buttock muscles to stay tight and contracted to keep the body erect to perform its function. Unfortunately, when the buttock muscles stay too tight for too long they can squeeze the nerve traveling underneath them called the sciatic nerve. When this happens the person will experience pain or dysfunction. In general, a postural irritation of sitting all day can lead to a functional irritation of pain.

The principals of the body follow the principals of natural law. An engineering principal called the piezoelectric effect states that a mass will remodel itself to the pressure put on it. When a wood beam is being placed in a weight bearing position supporting a house and the beam is receiving an uneven amount of weight bearing from on one end, it will bow or warp in response to that excessive weight. This same principal is applicable to the human frame and body. Imbalances from the structure including head tilt, shoulder height, spinal balance, hip, knee or ankle distortions redistribute weight bearing unevenly and eventually will create dysfunction.

The best way to avoid developmental structural conditions is to use prevention. Have your postural balance checked by a Chiropractor now so that you don't develop more functional problems later.

Quote of the week: *"If you don't understand yourself you don't understand anybody else."*—Nikki Giovanni

Super-size your meal—super-size your body

Question: My daughter is in high school and eats fast-food dinners after her evening soccer practices and games. I am trying to tell her that her weight problem is from these fast-food meals, especially when she super-sizes them. Is it rue these fast food meals contribute to her weight gain?

Answer: Fast food, excluding salads, is a major cause of obesity in our youth today. Without naming any specific multimillion dollar fast food chain, I can undoubtedly tell you that fast food is loaded with unhealthy saturated fats, dense carbohydrates and soaring sugar levels.

It isn't the fat or sugar that makes us gain weight as much as the dense carbohydrates that go undigested. Undigested carbohydrates are converted to fat in the body and this is what gives your daughter weight gain.

The super-sizing of meals for a small increase in price was a brilliant marketing scheme. It also has generated an even greater degree of weight problems for the consumer.

A group of concerned national public-advocates organization called the National Alliance for Nutrition and Activity (NANA) is collectively campaigning to stop "manipulation" of the consumer by the food industry. NANA believes that super-sizing for a bargain leads people to eat more food then they need or even want. They suggest that the public begin asking for smaller portions, half portions or share food with someone else.

Our nation, especially our youth, have a serious illness called obesity. The combination of record levels of fast-food consumption combined with diminished physical activity leads to rapid weight gain. It is not the early cosmetic damage a child lives with that a parent should be concerned with. The excess weight can lead to juvenile diabetes, joint dysfunction and heart and lung conditions.

My advice is to prepare health meals at home so your daughter breaks this dangerous habit.

Quote of the week: *"One loyal friend is worth 10,000 relatives."*—Euripides

Take control when it comes to kids' diets

Question: I am concerned my children are not getting enough nutritious food in their diet on a daily basis. What could I do to ensure they are getting the right amount of minerals and vitamins?

Answer: A parent has a constant struggle to get their children to eat correctly and nutritiously. Society is so fast paced that we get "too busy" to make sure our children eat appropriately. Eating habits outside the home are deplorable. I would not depend on our schools to guarantee healthy nutritious meals, either. When given a choice, a child will choose a cupcake over an apple. Making lunch for your child is a wise choice. Increase the amount of fiber, fresh fruit and vegetables at lunchtime, and you have begun to improve your child's diet.

Children love sugar. The average can of soda contains approximately 10 teaspoons of refined sugar. A four-ounce candy bar and a can of cola contain enough sugar to suppress the immune system for up to six hours. Ten teaspoons of sugar decrease your immune function by 50 percent, while 24 teaspoons decrease your immune system function by 92 percent.

Here are some more alarming statistics: The average American child consumes five pounds of sugar a week! By age 12, an estimated 70 percent of our children have developed the beginning stages of hardening of the arteries and are considered obese.

Nutrition plays a significant role in your child's health. The greater the amount of minerals and vitamins your child can digest, the greater their immune system will be enhanced. The national Cancer Institute and the American Heart Society both recommend five to nine servings of raw fruits and vegetables a day to prevent cancer, heart disease and strokes. Unfortunately, most fruits and vegetables loose 75 percent of their nutritional value within five days after being harvested. By the time they even get into the market, they could already be three to four days old.

There are some wonderful alternatives to assist you in maintenance of your children's diets. A product I have used with my own children is called Juice-Plus+, which comes in a gummy, chewable or capsule form. The gummies taste great and contain 17 raw fruits and veggies and two grains that will give your child a nutritional edge to assist their immune systems during this cold and flu season. For information visit www.juiceplus.com.

I believe there is no better substitute for a great nutritious diet than to literally eat a great nutritious diet. It is a little more work these days, so shop often, prepare ahead, and educate yourself on proper food combing.

Quote of the week: *"Problems are only opportunities in work clothes."*—Henry J. Kaiser

Therapy can help hypochondriacs

Question: My aunt always has something wrong with her. If it isn't her back, its headaches, stomach pain and many other symptoms. This is going on for over 15 years and I am convinced she is a hypochondriac. What can be done to help her?

Answer: Billions of dollars are spent by hypochondriacs on unnecessary diagnostic testing and doctor's visits yearly. According to Harvard Medical School research hypochondriacs run up medical cost 15 percent.

Many physicians feel these type patients need psychological help. A study by the American Psychosomatic Society indicated that group therapy reduced medical costs by over $1,000 for those who participated in group therapy versus those that did not.

Clinically, we predominately see a direct link between patients emotional experiences and physical sensations. Obviously, not all patients are hypochondriacs; in fact my belief is none are. Some people just need to find the correct treatment medium to help conquer their problems.

Long-term physical stress can lead to emotional distress and long term psychological stress can lead to physical ailments.

There are those patients that refuse to let go of their fears, pains and ailments. Many patients are their own worse enemy. I believe they must heal from within and spending enormous amounts of money on multitude of doctors is an expression of their inability to confront reality. Unfortunately, many of these patients end up on antidepressants. The drugs may help calm these patients and allow them to exist in society, but to be well someday they will have to combat themselves and let go.

Quote of the week: *"Victim of this, victim of that, your daddy's to thin and momma's too fat. Get over it!"*—Eagles

Thoracic-outlet syndromes respond to Chiropractic

Question: I have been diagnosed with thoracic-outlet syndrome. I get pain in my right arm that goes into my hands and fingers. My arms go numb at night, especially if I put them under my head to sleep. Is there anything a Chiropractor can do to help my condition?

Answer: Thoracic-outlet syndrome is a compression of the subclavian artery and or the brachial plexus nerves as they pass over your first rib and then under your clavicle and its overlying musculature. The entrapment of the blood vessels and the nerves in the lowest portion of your neck, where it meets your shoulders, is a very common irritation and a very serious condition.

The condition is affected by various factors. Vigorous work or muscular exercise may result in an increase of muscular bulk, thereby reducing the space through which the artery vein and nerves must pass. Congenital factors such as a cervical rib, or a bony protuberance on the first rib may cause pressure on the vessels or nerves when the arm is in certain positions. Traumatic causes of these syndromes are fractures of the clavicle and dislocations of the shoulder. A blood vessel exiting this thoracic area that is narrowed or sclerotic due to disease or aging can give these symptoms also.

In general, the symptoms consist of pain in the fingers, hand, forearm, arm, and shoulder along with abnormal sensations, felt along the back of the arm and hand. Numbness is also common in the fingers and in more severe cases coldness, weakness and discoloration.

Carpal-tunnel syndrome, which is entrapment of the median nerve and blood vessels, may be associated with thoracic-outlet syndromes but should be differentially diagnosed to avoid unnecessary surgery.

Thoracic-outlet syndrome responds well to Chiropractic treatment. Precise adjustments to the cervical and thoracic spine along with adjacent joints realigns structures to allow proper nerve and blood supply. Reduction of spasm and muscle inflammation also reduces irritation. In severe cases surgery may be necessary.

Quote of the week: *"Say what you mean, mean what you say, and do not be mean when you say it."*—Meryl Runion

Vegan diet is healthiest of all

Question: I have read a lot of your columns regarding the dreadful diets we have as Americans and how our children are obese. I understand the basics on how to eat correctly, but could you give me your opinion on the best and safest diet for my children and me?

Answer: The best and safest diet is the vegetarian diet. A vegan (totally vegetarian) diet is one that consists of eating absolutely no animal products and all naturally prepared foods. Ultimately these foods would be organic, unrefined, and unprocessed. Vegetarians have to be careful as omnivores with their food sources due to genetically manufactured food products, and the use of pesticides and fertilizers potentially contaminating their food.

The vegan diet can supply all necessary proteins, minerals, and vitamins that any other diet can perform. The vitamins that may not be as sufficient in a meat inclusive diet are some "B" vitamins, which can be supplemented by using nutritional yeast. When eating correctly and intelligently on a vegan diet your energy soars and your body is healthy with little or no illness. I have witnessed patient's skin conditions heal as well as countless other dramatic positive improvements in their health. Eating a vegetarian diet improperly can have the reverse effects of health by not understanding appropriate protein balancing and food combining. The old stereotype vegetarian was one that was excessively thin and sickly looking. Modern vegetarians make up many of our healthiest model citizens.

Eating a vegetarian diet is the easiest diet on the planet when you eat at home and it is becoming easier in public. Most fine restaurants and even diners offer vegetarian alternatives. Raw salads have become one of the number one lunch items even in the U.S. Thousands of books are available on vegetarianism as well as hundreds of web sites.

Reasons to become a vegetarian transcend just the personal health consideration. Most vegans I know have a very strong conviction about saving our planet and the animal's fortunate to still be left on it. Every vegetarian meal you eat saves an animal's life. Every vegetarian meal you eat allows our earth to regenerate new life. In ten years from now you may not have a choice to eat animals and may be forced to eat a predominantly or totally vegetarian diet. I believe the time is now and this method of food consumption is best and safest for you and your family.

As I have disclosed before, if we don't do anything about our children's diets now, one in three will have diabetes due to obesity in the year 2008. McDonald's recently refused to accept beef injected with antibiotics and hormones due to its terrible health effects. What do we do about all the contaminated beef that was consumed over the last 50 years? Mad cow disease, farmed seafood, SARS, and what next? You asked what is best, well vegan is the best!

Quote of the week: *"Animals are my friends, and I don't eat my friends."*—George Bernard Shaw

Vertigo and whiplash may be connected

Question: My mom has severe vertigo and has seen many specialists without any relief. The medications the physicians gave her did not help either. Recently she shared with me that her vertigo started about the same time her neck pain did. Is there a correlation between the two and can Chiropractic help?

Answer: Vertigo is defined as a sensation of dizziness. There are many causes of vertigo including inner ear disturbances, visual dysfunction, neurological disorders, and many more. As you have already discovered, getting an accurate diagnosis as well as an appropriate cure can be exhausting. Most modern medications are geared to give relief but fail to correct the cause as your mom has experienced. As Chiropractors we look to the cause of the condition by looking at the source of nerve supply to the malfunctioning tissue involved. It may not have been a coincidence your mother's neck pain occurred around the same time her vertigo did. There is direct nerve supply from the cervical nerve roots into the eyes, ears, nose, throat, and entire cranial region. A disruption of the nerve supply to any of these areas could have a direct or indirect effect on the sensation of dizziness.

In my Chiropractic practice many patients complain of vertigo upon their initial consultation. I have found that this is a common symptom secondary to a whiplash type injury to the neck area. It has also been clinically evident as the neck condition improves so does the symptom of vertigo. You should not take vertigo lightly. Although many patients respond well to Chiropractic adjustments, there is a chance that a more severe underlying condition exists. Persistent or progressive irritation of the vertigo may require extensive diagnostic testing including a brain computerized tomography (CT) scan, magnetic-resonance imaging (MRI), and nerve testing. Our philosophy is to start with conservative care and proceed only if no progress is made or symptoms increase.

Quote of the week: *"He who overcomes others is strong, but he who overcomes himself is mightier."*—John Henry Patterson

Visualization therapy can combat illness

Question: I am a cancer survivor and utilized visual therapy to heal. Can using this therapy enhance spinal corrections?

Answer: I personally am a strong advocate of conceptual/visual therapy. Many Chiropractors and other healers simultaneously utilize the same principals like you as a patient. Your brain can be programmed to respond to conditions. Installing programs that reverse detrimental illness are very real and successful methods of combating mental and physical illness.

Conceptual healing educates the patients to see themselves as healing or totally free of their disease state. It is not the cure by any means and should never be substituted for appropriate medical or Chiropractic treatment. We can convince the body and mind to enhance it's responses to the healing process by visualizing each step of the healing process in a clear, precise, active state. The more specific and educated the patient is in their conceptualizing, the more effective they can create the re-patterning and improvement of their condition. An example is a cervical spine whiplash patient who would envision increased mobility in their cervical vertebrae, soft, flexible smooth, contracting neck muscles with a warm flow of gentle calmness to the surrounding soft tissue. The greater the amount of these senses utilized the more effective in assisting the brain and treatment.

Your Chiropractor can enhance the effect of their treatment to you by envisioning the same result, as they adjust your spine.

What you can conceive, you can achieve. How you see yourself and how you feel can be a mirror image. Take a chance, look at your reflection and start looking at yourself as healthy. It just might happen.

Quote of the week: *"There can be no happiness if the things we believe in are different from the things we do."*—Freya Madeline Stack

Vitamin supplement content can be deceiving

Question: I take a lot of vitamin supplements yet I don't feel I am getting the benefits from them. What makes one vitamin supplement better than another?

Answer: The Food and Drug Administration presently has loose restrictions on vitamin manufacturers' labels.

The loose restrictions are that contents are listed but absorption rates and the ability to breakdown the supplement after digested are not listed. The outer coating, nor how the supplement is (adhering) to form its shape are not always listed. Many less effective supplements are produced with glucose (sugar) coatings which give the shiny appearance to the exterior surface. In these supplements breakdown and absorption will unlikely not occur in the gut wall where most of the benefit occurs. Multi-vitamins classically are produced in this manner. Sugar or carbohydrate type coatings can also be very allergic to many people, not only preventing nutritional value but also irritating the stomach.

The closer to natural food the supplements is the greater its absorption and nutritional value. Avoid supplements with sugars, food colorings, artificial ingredients and that may be allergenic

Nutritionists, Chiropractors and Homeopathic Physicians have training in nutrition and can guide you to appropriate supplementation, if needed.

The best way to get great nutritional supplementation is to eat properly and you will not need vitamin supplements at all.

Quote of the week: *"The indispensable first step to getting the things you want of life is this, decide what you want."*—Ben Stein

Well patient need not get an adjustment

Question: I recently went to my Chiropractor because I was feeling sick with a fever, runny nose and congestion. After he analyzed my spine he didn't adjust me at all and said I was balanced and clear. Why would he do this?

Answer: Congratulations! You demonstrated just how self-healing the human body could be. The confusion you are having is in your definition of sickness. The beginning of symptoms, what we have always called "sickness," is really your body getting well. Traditional medical thinking calls the presence of symptoms "sickness." The truth is you are sick before the onset of your symptoms. The symptoms are really an indication that your body has accurately recognized an invader or toxin and is actively responding to it by creating a fever, mucous cough, diarrhea, vomiting etc., to eliminate it from your body. A symptom is a protective mechanism of the body to alert it something is out of control. It is the last line of protection to show up and the first to go away. Covering up symptoms with medication can interrupt natural functions of healing.

Did you ever ask yourself why a fever occurs in the body? One of the main reasons is to create an environment that kills bacteria or viruses. The brilliant innate intelligence of the human body is built to be perfect. Being conscious of our body's directives and having faith in you ability to heal allows a person to accept that many common symptoms that you call "sickness" are welcome healthy functions of the body.

When your Chiropractor decided not to adjust you he/she was acknowledging the wisdom of the body and supporting wellness rather than sickness. Sacrificing temporary relief to feel better using medications is discarding the big picture, which is allowing the body to naturally function through natural elimination and self-healing. Your Chiropractor trusted that your balanced nervous system, which controls all other tissue healing directly and indirectly, could satisfy the task of maintaining your wellness.

There is a difference between getting sick and getting well. Know to trust your body and allow the natural process of healing to occur when it needs it. And finally, make sure you continue to live you life in a way that not only prevents sickness, but also creates health, happiness and wholeness.

Quote of the week: *"Trusting our intuition often saves us from disaster."*—Anne Wilson Shaef

Well-rested children are healthier

Question: I have two elementary-school children that want to stay up late, even on school nights. Is it true that staying up late at their ages is unhealthy and stressful? Please verify if this is true or not.

Answer: I emphasize with your predicament regarding late-night bedtime for elementary school-age children. I have two boys myself and must battle to get them to bed early every school night. The answer to this for your children and my children and every other parent that has the same concern is yes, early to bed children fair better emotionally and physiologically. A study done at Brown University Medical School gave 138 third grade girls stressful tasks during a few hours spent at their homes. The researchers measured initial levels of the stress hormone cortisol in saliva samples and rechecked cortisol after each task. The girls' weeknight bedtimes correlated with their stress hormone response. Those going to bed early released more cortisol after the first stressful experience, but compared with girls kept up past 9 p.m., their stress hormones declined more steeply during the next two tasks. Kids with later bedtimes, were more uncomfortable during the tasks than the children who got more sleep.

Prolonged output of cortisol can raise blood pressure and heart rate; weaken immune response, so that colds and other viruses take hold more easily; and make it harder to concentrate when challenged.

The findings apply to boys as well as girls. The study also found preliminary evidence of nervous system changes in sleep-deprived children. Children's sleep needs vary and the majority can handle mild degrees of sleep depravations, but some do just terribly.

It can sometimes be stressful just putting your children to bed at the appropriate time. I personally would rather deal with an upset child at bedtime than a cranky child in the morning, especially when attempting to meet deadlines as well as making sure the children eat a healthy breakfast.

I agree with you that a parent's responsibility is to get their child to bed at a reasonable time and to maintain a consistency in that time to reduce stress and maintain a healthy nervous system.

Quote of the week: *"Experience…is simply the name we give our mistakes."*—Oscar Wilde

You can lose weight in a healthy way

Question: I recently did this fad diet and lost a lot of weight but I feel worse than ever. Is losing weight supposed to make you ill?

Answer: Fad diets and quick weight loss schemes are dangerous and can make you ill or even kill you. Rapid weight loss breaks down muscle as opposed to fat and changes your body composition producing increased risk to other serious health concerns.

Unhealthy body composition increases the risk of developing high-blood pressure, high cholesterol, cardiovascular disease, insulin insensitivity, type two diabetes, hormone imbalances and more.

A healthy body composition program helps a person weigh less and look thinner by causing excess fat to be lost and muscle to be retained. Healthy body composition produces significantly better overall health.

America is in a state of health emergency. More than 60 percent of the U.S. Adult population is overweight, and more than 25 percent are considered obese. One out of four children and adolescents are now considered overweight or obese and are quickly headed for a lifetime of chronic disease.

We are fatter than ever and the number continues to rise at a dreadfully high rate. Even more alarming is the fact that approximately 20 percent of the overweight Americans may not realize they need to lose excess body fat, because they physically "appear" to be normal weight. Despite looking thin and having a normal weight, they have altered or unhealthy body composition.

Achieving healthy body composition is critically important to experiencing the joy that optimal health can bring. You have the power to shape your body for better health. Discuss healthy diets and lifestyles with your Chiropractor to find the best approach catered to your individual needs.

Quote of the week: *"Life is only a comparison of who we are with who we would rather be."*—Author unknown

What is better — bottled or tap water?

Question: I know I am supposed to drink eight glasses of water a day, but the kind of water I should drink is very confusing. What do you suggest?

Answer: According to a group that studies water called Co-op America as much as 40 percent of bottled water is actually bottled tap water, sometimes with additional treatments, sometimes not. Bottled water is a monstrous industry. Americans paid $77 billion for bottled water in 2002 according the consulting and research firm Beverage Marketing Corp.

There is an environmental issue with bottled water because 90 percent of water bottles end up as either garbage or litter at a rate of 30 million bottles a day. Potentially toxic additives along with chlorine are released into the air from their incineration.

Bottled water may not be safer than tap water according to some studies. There are regulations in most municipalities for water but many other studies have shown higher risk of certain diseases when regularly consuming city tap water. To combat the potential toxic exposure to contaminated or infected city water I suggest a home charcoal or reverse osmosis water filtration which will leave your water pure and tasting great. When you are on the road use bottled water that you have verified to truly be pure.

Your exclusive beverage should be water and yes, eight glasses a day is essential to maintain optimum health. It is best to drink water at room temperature.

Avoid distilled water since it has the wrong ionization, pH, polarization and oxidation potentials. It will also drain your body of minerals.

I also suggest you avoid purchasing the one-gallon cloudy plastic (PVC) containers from your grocery store since they transfer too many chemicals into the water. The five-gallon containers and the ones in the clear bottles (polythylene) are a much better plastic and will not give the water a plastic taste.

To assure purity, call the water company selling it and get an "independent lab assessment" of water quality and stick with companies that can provide this information.

Quote of the week: *"In helping others we shall help ourselves, for whatever good we give out completes the circle and comes back to us."*—Hora Edwards

Closing metaphorical stories — a great way to segue with new patients

The story of wild geese

When you see geese heading south for the winter flying along in the "V" formation, you might be interested in knowing what science has discovered about why they fly that way. As each bird flaps its wings, it creates uplift for the bird immediately following. By flying in a "V" formation, the whole flock adds at least 71-percent greater flying range than if each bird flew on its own. This is quite similar to people who are part of a team and share a common direction to get where they are going quicker and easier, because they are traveling on the trust of one another and lift each other up along the way.

Whenever a goose falls out of formation, it suddenly feels the drag and resistance of trying to go through it alone and quickly gets back into formation to take advantage of the power of the flock. If we have as much sense as a goose, we will stay in formation and share information with those who are headed the same way that we are going.

When the lead goose gets tired, it rotates back in the wing and another goose takes over. It pays to share leadership and take turns doing hard jobs. The geese honk from behind to encourage those up front to keep their speed. Words of support and inspiration help energize those on the front line, helping them to keep pace in spite of the day-to-day pressures and fatigue. It is important that our honking be encouraging. Otherwise it's just — well ... honking!

Finally, when a goose gets sick or is wounded by a gunshot and falls out, two geese fall out of the formation and follow the injured one down to help and protect it. They stay with it until he is either able to fly or dead. Then they launch out with another formation to catch up with their group. When one of us is down, it's up to the others to stand by us in our time of trouble. If we have the sense of a goose, we will stand by each other when things get rough. We will stay in formation with those headed where we want to go.

The next time you see a formation of geese, remember their message that — it is indeed a reward, a challenge and a privilege to be a contributing member of a team.

Author unknown

Attitudes are more important than facts

There was a beginning teacher in Illinois who fell in love with teaching during her first year in the classroom. Because the school principal had not visited her classroom to evaluate her teaching skills, she assumed that she would not be employed the following year. At the end of the school year she took her materials to the office and prepared to say good-bye.

The principal saw her and said, We have enjoyed having you here this year and look forward to having you teach with us again next year."

She was quite surprised and replied, "Well, I haven't received a contract to teach next year, so I just assumed you thought I had done a poor job and didn't want me back."

The principal said, "We really want you back. Your students have scored higher on their achievement tests than any of our other students in the last 10 years. You've got to come back next year."

The teacher said, "It's easy to teach when you have such a great group of kids as I had. They were sharp, interested, motivated, and all of them had IQs of 150, 152, 153 and even higher."

The principal asked how she knew that the students had such high IQ scores. She mentioned the materials he had given her at the beginning of the school year, which contained a sheet of paper with the students' names and IQ scores on it.

He smiled at her and said, "Those were their locker numbers."

Because she thought the students had high IQ scores, she had treated them all year as if they did. Her attitude was one of high expectations. She believed in the students. She knew they could accomplish the work. Her experience underscores the point that "attitudes are more important than facts."

Art Gardner
"Why Winners Win"

Polar bear cages

In the Northern parts of Alaska polar bears are attracted to the city dwellings by the scents of food. The bears leave the back woods country and travel to the outskirts of the cities where they keep large dumpsters of garbage. The strength and size of the polar bears is too much to prevent them from overturning the large metal garbage dumpsters.

The problem is that if these polar bears receive their meals from the garbage without hunting they quickly become accustomed to the free food and loose their natural instinct to hunt on their own.

To prevent this behavior game wardens and animal control authorities will tag the polar bears and/or spray paint their white fur with bright orange numbers to track their activities. Should the polar bears return to the garbage site they are placed 5 to 10 miles away. If they return a third time it is indicative of a loss of natural hunting instinct and they must be destroyed or put in a zoo.

This one particular polar bear was caught for his third time at the garbage dump. Fortunately for him a brand new zoo was opening in Denver, Colorado. The animal control authorities built him a large 12' by 12' cage to transport him to Colorado. When the polar bear got in the cage he paced back and forth, 12' in one direction to the end of the cage and then 12' in the opposite direction to the end of the cage.

Due to red tape and lack of funding there was a delay in the opening of the zoo. The polar bear was stuck, confined to his cage to pace 12' in one direction and then 12' in the other direction, for 8 months.

Finally, after 8 months of pacing 12' in one direction and 12' in the opposite direction, the zoo opened. It was a natural habitat zoo and the visitors felt they were observing the animals in a naturally beautifully landscaped environment. With much pomp and circumstance the exciting day had come to lift the 12' by 12' cage with the polar bear into his new natural habitat by crane. The crane lowered the cage into the habitat and unloaded the polar bear, lifting the empty cage up and away.

What do you think the polar bear did? He paced 12' in one direction and 12' in the other direction, even without the confines of the physical cage restricting him.

The metaphor of the story is: We all have invisible polar bear cages that we created over time. Behavioral habits are existing whether you can see them or not. Every once in a while we have an opportunity to break a non-productive habit and travel outside our polar bear cage. Chiropractic is the solution to your new freedom. Take this opportunity and run to unlimited health and happiness.

Stories of inspiration…from the heart

Speaking engagement snafus

I started my career as a Chiropractor with fearless passion to educate every person I met with the miracles that Chiropractic offers. There wasn't any person anywhere I wouldn't tell the Chiropractic story to. One of my first patients was a nurse at what she described as an elderly home. She offered me an opportunity to give my first outside-the-office speaking engagement at the elderly home. I was thrilled to be able to speak to a group of people.

I practiced my talk over and over until I could repeat it in my sleep. I chose the topic of exercise and the elderly. Of course I would finish with my Chiropractic story. I made a checklist of posters, models, and hand-outs. I was bursting with excitement over the expectations of the first of what would be more than 1,000 public lectures. I was soon to learn first meant initial as in initiation.

My patient's vague description of the elderly home became clearer as I entered the building. It wasn't quite an elderly home as she described. It was a convalescent hospital with critically ill elderly patients, all of whom had anywhere from weeks to months to live. I met my nurse patient just prior to entering the room and she apologized for not telling me the truth about the presentation. She said she didn't think I would come if I knew the degree of illnesses her patients had. This only pumped me up more because I was in the save-the-world mode and was ready. Or was I?

I set my tripod up with lecture posters and organized my materials. When I turned around to face the audience I noticed they were all in wheel chairs, many of them with portable IVs attached. Directly to my left was an elderly woman about arm's length away. Before I could speak "hello" she cursed at me as loud as her lungs could bear. She continued to curse at me for an entire half-hour. I heard curses I never knew existed. It ended up she had a condition called Tourette's Syndrome, which is characterized by uncontrollable outbreaks of profanity. Immediately to my right was an elderly gentleman who had Parkinson's disease, which included a repetitive twitch of his head that caused him to spew, spit in my direction. So, before I even spoke a word I had a woman cursing loudly on my left and a man spitting on me on my right.

My topic was exercise and the elderly. I managed to get through about half the talk, when unfortunately one of the patients coded and had to be rushed out of the room for emergency life resuscitation. Never forgetting my mission I somehow focused on completing my talk. There were four other nurses in the room during my lecture. They got such a kick out of the heckling and distractions and my perseverance to get my message across that they all signed up to be new patients and are still my patients to this day.

Since that first initiation I have learned that talks never go as expected and that is why I love the challenge of speaking.

A mother's testimony — breech technique successful in turning twins

My name is Cindy. I'm a mother of a 14-year-old and a 4-year-old, both boys, and I am currently pregnant with fraternal twin boys.

I have been receiving Chiropractic care for the past 15 years and have my family receiving Chiropractic care too. I'm a fairly new patient of Steven Pollack, DC, and have been completely satisfied with his treatment. But, there is one treatment that totally surprised me and one that I'll always be grateful for.

During this twin pregnancy, I had a few complications. One particular one was that between my 30th and 34th week of pregnancy the twin on the bottom (baby "B") was sitting butt down or breech for too long. My doctors said that the baby would probably not turn because of his size and there was little room, and I would have to be scheduled for a Cesarean section, while my other children were born natural, this surgery concerned me a lot.

At a regular visit with Dr. Pollack, I told him of the situation. He said he knew of an adjustment that might turn the baby and it may take one or two treatments. To tell you the truth I was a little skeptical that the baby would actually turn, but I had no problem trying the adjustment.

The next day I had an appointment for a sonogram. The babies had gained weight and would you believe, baby "B" had turned, head down at 35 weeks!

I was genuinely amazed and very happy. This was the best fit I received throughout my entire pregnancy. As it stands we are just waiting for the babies, and anticipate an exciting natural twin birth.

When I returned to Dr. Pollack's office, I told him what had happened. We were both so thrilled that we hugged each other. I couldn't be more thankful and grateful for what he did for me and my family. I truly believe in Chiropractic care and go regularly. I will not miss the opportunity to experience a natural twin birth.

Thank you Dr. Pollack.

By Cindy Stallone

Paying tribute to a hero

We have come to define heroes in America as people who have braved difficult circumstances, sacrificed themselves to benefit others and served for a purpose that was pure and unadulterated.

On Tuesday, August 6, one of my heroes passed away. Her name was Cheryl Jean Pasciak. Cheryl Jean and her parents personify the term hero.

For six years of her life, Cheryl Jean fought leukemia. She never gave up even in her last breath. This 10-year-old little angel on earth cherished every second of every day. She managed to give smiles for everyone she met even with her body and insides screaming in pain. Cheryl Jean displaced her won personal turmoil by redirecting her attention on helping others feel better. She didn't know this consciously, but it was obvious.

We all should learn from the lessons Cheryl Jean was teaching us. Cherish every moment and consider others first.

For Cheryl Jean's parents, it was six years of unconditional love. We sometimes forget about the caretaker of these children going through the battle. I wish to acknowledge Linda and John for demonstrating to me the true meaning of unconditional love. They sacrificed everything to make their child's every moment on this planet more comfortable. In doing so, they created a bond that many parents can only dream about.

These two exemplify the relationship we all could have with our kids if we put our heart and soul into it. They may have lost their daughter after 10 years, but the bond they had with her will last an eternity. I thank them for reminding me how short life is and how every moment with your children should be quality time, not just occasionally.

Heroes exist to set the bar just a little higher in our own lives. Heroes give us personality traits to emulate. I will miss Cheryl Jean's bear hugs, but I will remember her every time I see someone and smile. Part of that smile will belong to Cheryl Jean.

Quote of the week: *"When I call your name, would you be the same, if I see you in heaven?"*—Eric Clapton

I survived an avalanche

Buried alive under 15 feet of snow is not what my epitaph will read. My time wasn't up yet, and I didn't hear any fat lady singing.

On Tuesday, March 5, 1991 I went helicopter skiing at Whistler-Black-home ski area in Western Canada. The previous two days left the mountains with two feet of fresh, deep powder. Endless ice glaciers created the back bowls of the mountains. The snow was five feet deep in most spots. It is a dream for skiers to experience deep powder skiing and some have equaled it to an orgasm.

It wasn't for lack of an orgasm that I scheduled my trip. I love adventure, challenge, and living on the edge. These are pre-requirements for heli-skiing.

Our group was made up of 10 along with a guide. There was Carol and Ian, cabin attendants for British Airways from London; Hans, a Swedish loner out for fun; Tony, an experienced Canadian heli-skier with more than 100 trips under his belt; Joe and Marcia, a general surgeon and his wife from Boston; and finally myself, a Chiropractor and my two close fiends, Dave and Ulysis, both Neurologists. Our pre-ski instructions included how to prepare runaway straps for lost skis in deep powder. They were bright fluorescent orange and ran about 1½ feet in length while attaching to the ski brakes and tucked into the ski boot. Our next demonstration was on how to utilize avalanche beepers. They are basically turned on and never touched unless there is a rare chance of an avalanche, at which time everyone above ground turns theirs off so the buried beeper attached to the snow-covered person can be isolated. Final instructions are given on helicopter safety. Skis are never to be held vertically and you don't lift your head up around the one-ton blades traveling at 50-miles an hour.

The helicopter ride starts the adrenaline pumping. The view of the vast snow-covered glacier is astounding. Snow engulfed mountains can be seen in all 360 degrees. We landed on a mountaintop, exiting quickly and gathering our skis and poles. The helicopter left us there. The only way down now is to ski, or at least that's what you would suspect. Our guide points to a spot to meet, about 1,000 feet below us. The snow is amazingly deep, almost waist height. It's slow moving and difficult to turn. I am used to Eastern ice and hard-pack conditions. This is totally different. Each movement I make is deliberate and slow motion. My mind is playing the pictures I read in a magazine on how to ski the powder. Skis together to make a single foundation, turn wide and slowly, weight forward, and lift the body up at the end of each turn. I embarrassingly fell twice before we even reached the first bowl. At this point I was excited and determined to conquer nature's challenge of deep-powder skiing, leaving new tracks, and figure eighths behind me. Unfortunately I never got that chance. Our guide determined he would be the first one down the first bowl. After he reached the bottom, each skier would follow one by one, waiting until the bottom was reached. The guide went first and it looked great. Next Marcia, next Joe, then David started down. Ulysis and I moved to the center on the bowl at its peak, more than 850 feet. We watched as David made slow hop turns. He was halfway down when a thunderous rattle occurred, engulfing the entire bow. Our first instinct was that it was just a noise, thunder maybe. Our minds were initially in denial similar to the first stage of realization in death. Simultaneously with the thunder came a shaking of the snow and earth beneath our feet. Time stood still. It couldn't be happening. Our temporary stupor was aroused when the guide at the very bottom of the mountain yelled up AVALANCHE! Reality set in.

My friend Ulysis, an emotionally solid, brilliant, stable doctor from North Jersey lost it.

In his Argentinean accent, which he rarely uses, he cried out, "Steve, Steve, we are going to die. It's all over. This is it!"

Usually the vocal one, I was speechless. I could not conjure up even a vowel sound. The moments before the entire mountain gave way were in slow motion. We definitely knew what was happening but could not stop our fate. We were helpless. As the denial turned into a sharper reality in my mind, so many thoughts ran through my head simultaneously that it all became a blur. Then the entire earth rose 3 to 4 feet, similar to the effect of an earthquake. It was like a powerful wave at the beach. We were riveted off balance and sucked below the avalanching snow…falling, rolling, tumbling deeper and deeper. I felt my emotions leave and enter the final stage of death—acceptance.

I was rolling with this huge wave. There was no conception of time or space. Everything was bright white and clear. The rolling effect was returning me to the comfort of the womb. At this point I accepted my fate and was totally at peace, no thoughts, just a spiritual experience. This was "it." The movement slowed down temporarily and I knew I was approximately 15 to 20 feet deep under the snow.

Just as soon as it slowed down there came a second powerful wave of bursting force. It awoke me out of my passive complacency. I jolted my chest forward and arched my neck up. This innate action was the source of my survival. I shot toward the surface like a bullet and then the movement stopped. The pressure from the snow piled up and started to compress my back, neck, ribs, and legs. The squeeze on my body was tremendous. Then this stopped.

I was still breathing and I was buried under the snow. I was totally disoriented. I didn't know which was up or down, nor where I was. In less than a minute I heard the voice of Ulysis. This time his voice was sharp and clear. It was above me. Looking toward the sound, I arched my neck up and saw lighter, brighter snow. I moved my head up and forced it to the surface. I broke through the surface of the snow taking in a deep breath of crisp fresh air while squinting at the sunshine. I saw the light, no more darkness, no more fright. Never had air or sunlight meant so much to me.

We take so much for granted. There was Ulysis, just three feet away from me. He was almost at arm's distance away. We were alive and saved. I wiggled the rest of my body out of the snow. It was covered about four feet deep on a slant. I sat up and contemplated returning from my lapse of unconsciousness. I literally pinched myself and spoke. It was true. I survived.

We lost our skis on the initial fall and one ski edge sliced open my right knee requiring 17 sutures. Bazaar parts of my outfit had been ripped off — zippers, buttons, straps, etc. The avalanche was the worse in British Columbia in 20 years. We had fallen more than 850 feet. No one died.

My friend Dave, who was halfway down the mountain when the avalanche started, was buried six feet under — still wearing his skis. By divine luck we heard his muffled yells for help, even with his face down in the snow.

One side note. While sitting up I noticed my right hand was clenched around my ski pole. I had to deliberately let my fingers off one by one. I believe subconsciously I did this knowing that it would be a last salvation to poke holes through the snow to find an air passage.

Life is dear and precious. My attitude toward life has always been to cherish each individual day. Now I am living on time granted to me by pre-destiny. I believe it wasn't my time to go the great beyond. You can buy material possessions but you can't buy time. Time is the most precious commodity on earth. I now treat every moment of every day as a special treat. Every day is my birthday. Life can be shorter and faster than we expect. A couple of old cliches come to mind: "Be here now" and "Love life itself."

0-595-32404-5